# SUGAR FREE . . . GOODIES

By Judith Soley Majors

### Cover Design
### Carrie Ann Majors

Apple Press
5536 S.E. Harlow
Milwaukie, Oregon  97222

Library of Congress Catalog Card Number: 89-070318

ISBN: 9-941905-00-4
Published by: Apple Press
              5536 S.E. Harlow
              Milwaukie, Oregon 97222

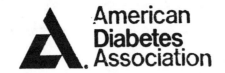
December 8, 1986

"Sugar Free...Goodies"

With the approval of the
American Diabetes Association, Inc.
Hawaii Affiliate, Inc.

*Jane K. Kadohiro*

Jane K. Kadohiro, RN, PHN
President

"Sugar Free . . . Goodies" is dedicated to the "sweet tooth" and good health of all those on special diets.

Judy Majors

and

To Carrie,

With much love and thanks for all of your help.

Mom

With very special heartfelt thanks to:

Jane Kadohiro, R.N. P.H.N., President, Hawaii Affiliate, technical assistance and coordination.

Sheila Beckham, R.D., M.P.H., technical assistance.

American Diabetes Association, Inc., Hawaii Affiliate, Inc., technical assistance.

Carrie Majors, production.

My family, never ending love and support.

# EXCHANGE LISTS

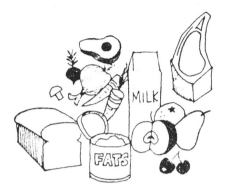

## EXCHANGE PROGRAM

The exchange program offers a variety of food to fit each individual's likes and needs in specific amounts. By using the six exchange lists and foods in specified numbers and amounts to fit your diet, you can create a variety of taste sensations and almost forget you're on a diet!

The exchange program is simply a trade of one food for another in a specific food group for a food that is nearly equal in calories, carbohydrates, protein and fat. Also foods in each exchange group have similar mineral and vitamin content.

A well balanced diet consists of foods from each food group, as no single exchange group can supply all the nutrients our body requires for good health.

The energy value of food is expressed by the calorie count. The primary energy sources are fats, proteins and carbohydrates. Sugars and starches are the most common carbohydrates. The foods in the following exchange lists work together to provide the necessary nutrients that are essential to body function.

The real trick is to carefully measure the amounts of food used. All amounts are given in household measurement and are based on the "new" ADA exchange lists.

5

## LIST 1
# STARCH/BREAD EXCHANGES

Each item in this list contains approximately 15 grams of carbohydrate, 3 grams of protein, a trace of fat, and 80 calories.

Whole grain products average about 2 grams of fiber per serving. Some foods are higher in fiber.

You can choose your starch servings from any of the items on this list. If you want to eat a starch food that is not on this list, the general rule is:

• 1/2 cup of cereal, grain, or pasta is one serving
• 1 ounce of a bread product is one serving

Your dietitian can help you be more exact.

### CEREALS/GRAINS/PASTA

| | |
|---|---|
| Bran cereals*, concentrated (such as Bran Buds®, All Bran®) | |
| Bran cereals, flaked | ½ cup |
| Bulgur (cooked) | ½ cup |
| Cooked cereals | ½ cup |
| Cornmeal (dry) | 2-½ tablespoons |
| Cornstarch | 2 tablespoons |
| Flour | 2-½ tablespoons |
| Grape nuts® | 3 tablespoons |
| Grits (cooked) | ½ cup |
| Other ready-to-eat unsweetened cereals | ¾ cup |
| Pasta (cooked) | ½ cup |
| Puffed cereal | 1-½ cups |
| Rice, white or brown (cooked) | ⅓ cup |
| Shredded wheat | ½ cup |
| Wheat germ* | 3 tablespoons |
| Wun tun pi | 6 tablespoons |

### DRIED BEANS, PEAS/LENTILS

| | |
|---|---|
| Barley, dry | 1-½ tablespoons |
| Beans* and peas* (cooked), such as kidney, white, split, blackeye | ⅓ cup |
| Baked beans* | ¼ cup |
| Lentils* | ⅓ cup |

### BREAD

| | |
|---|---|
| Bagel | ½ (1 ounce) |
| Bread sticks, crisp, 4 inches long x ½ inch wide | 2 (⅔ ounce) |
| Croutons, low-fat | 1 cup |
| English muffin | ½ |
| Frankfurter or hamburger bun | ½ (1 ounce) |
| Pita, 6 inches across | ½ |
| Plain roll, small | 1 (1 ounce) |
| Raisin, unfrosted | 1 slice (1 ounce) |
| Rye*, pumpernickel* | 1 slice (1 ounce) |
| Tortilla, 6 inches across | 1 |
| White (including French, Italian) | 1 slice (1 ounce) |
| Whole wheat | 1 slice (1 ounce) |

### CRACKERS/SNACKS

| | |
|---|---|
| Animal crackers | 8 |
| Graham crackers, 2-½-inch square | 3 |
| Matzo | ¾ ounce |
| Melba toast | 5 slices |
| Oyster crackers | 24 |
| Popcorn (popped, no fat added) | 3 cups |
| Pretzels | ¾ ounce |
| Rye crisp, 2 inches x 3-½ inches | 4 |
| Saltine-type crackers | 6 |
| Whole wheat crackers, no fat added (crisp breads, such as Finn®, Kavli®, Wasa®) | 2-4 slices (¾ ounce) |

## STARCH FOODS PREPARED WITH FAT
(Count as 1 Starch/Bread serving, plus 1 Fat serving)

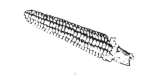

| | |
|---|---|
| Biscuit, 2-½ inches across | 1 |
| Chow mein noodles | ½ cup |
| Corn bread, 2-inch cube | 1 (2 ounces) |
| Cracker, round butter type | 6 |
| French fried potatoes, 2 to 3-½ inches long | 10 (1-½ ounces) |
| Muffin, plain, small | 1 |
| Pancake, 4 inches across | 2 |
| Stuffing, bread (prepared) | ¼ cup |
| Taco shell, 6 inches across | 2 |
| Waffle, 4-½-inch square | 1 |
| Whole wheat crackers, fat added (such as Triscuits©) | 4-6 (1 ounce) |

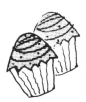

*400 milligrams or more of sodium per serving.

*3 grams or more of fiber per serving.

## STARCHY VEGETABLES

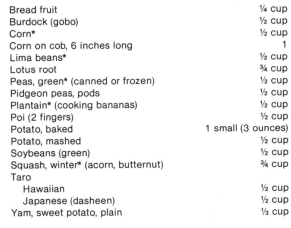

| | |
|---|---|
| Bread fruit | ¼ cup |
| Burdock (gobo) | ½ cup |
| Corn* | ½ cup |
| Corn on cob, 6 inches long | 1 |
| Lima beans* | ½ cup |
| Lotus root | ¾ cup |
| Peas, green* (canned or frozen) | ½ cup |
| Pidgeon peas, pods | ½ cup |
| Plantain* (cooking bananas) | ½ cup |
| Poi (2 fingers) | ½ cup |
| Potato, baked | 1 small (3 ounces) |
| Potato, mashed | ½ cup |
| Soybeans (green) | ½ cup |
| Squash, winter* (acorn, butternut) | ¾ cup |
| Taro | |
|     Hawaiian | ½ cup |
|     Japanese (dasheen) | ½ cup |
| Yam, sweet potato, plain | ⅓ cup |

## LIST 2
# MEAT EXCHANGES

The meat exchange list is divided into three parts based on the amount of fat and calories: Lean Meat, Medium-Fat Meat, and High-Fat Meat. One ounce (1 Meat Exchange) of each of these includes:

| | Carbohydrate (grams) | Protein (grams) | Fat (grams) | Calories |
|---|---|---|---|---|
| Lean | 0 | 7 | 3 | 55 |
| Medium-Fat | 0 | 7 | 5 | 75 |
| High-Fat | 0 | 7 | 8 | 100 |

You are encouraged to use more lean and medium-fat meat, poultry, and fish in your meal plan. This will help decrease your fat intake. You should try to limit your choices from the high-fat group to three times per week. Meat and substitutes do not contribute any fiber to your meal plan.

### LEAN MEAT AND SUBSTITUTES
(One Exchange is equal to any one of the following items.)

| | | |
|---|---|---|
| Beef: | USDA good or choice grades of lean beef, such as round, sirloin, flank steak, tenderloin, chipped beef*. | 1 ounce |
| Pork: | Lean pork, such as fresh ham; canned, cured or boiled ham*; Canadian bacon*; tenderloin | 1 ounce |
| Veal: | All cuts are lean except for veal cutlets (ground or cubed). Examples of lean veal are chops and roasts | 1 ounce |
| Poultry: | Chicken, turkey, Cornish hen (without skin) | 1 ounce |
| Fish: | All fresh and frozen fish | 1 ounce |
| | Crab, lobster, scallops, shrimp, clams* (fresh, or canned in water) | ounce (¼ cup) |
| | Oysters | 3 ounces (5 to 7 medium) |
| | Tuna* (canned in water) | ¼ cup |
| | Herring (uncreamed or smoked) | 1 ounce |
| | Sardines (canned) | 2 medium |
| Wild Game: | Venison, rabbit, squirrel | 1 ounce |
| | Pheasant, duck, goose (without skin) | 1 ounce |
| Cheese: | Any cottage cheese | ¼ cup |
| | Grated parmesan | 2 tablespoons |
| | Diet cheeses* with less than 55 calories per ounce | 1 ounce |
| Other: | 95 percent fat-free luncheon meat* | 1 ounce |
| | Egg whites | 3 whites |
| | Egg substitutes with less than 55 calories per ¼ cup | ¼ cup |

*400 milligrams or more of sodium per serving.
*3 grams or more of fiber per serving.

When purchasing meat, allow 4 ounces of raw meat for a 3 ounce cooked portion. For poultry with skin and bones allow an extra 1-½ – 2 ounces for skin and bones in a 4 ounce serving.

8

## MEDIUM-FAT MEAT AND SUBSTITUTES

(One exchange is equal to any one of the following items.)

| | | |
|---|---|---|
| *Beef:* | Most beef products fall into this category. Examples are: all ground beef, roast (rib, chuck, rump), steak (cubed, Porterhouse, T-bone), and meatloaf | 1 ounce |
| *Pork:* | Most pork products fall into this category. Examples are: chops, loin roast, Boston butt, cutlets. | 1 ounce |
| *Lamb:* | Most lamb products fall into this category. Examples are: chops, leg, and roast | 1 ounce |
| *Veal:* | Cutlet (ground or cubed, unbreaded) | 1 ounce |
| *Poultry:* | Chicken (with skin), domestic duck or goose (well-drained of fat), ground turkey | 1 ounce |
| *Fish:* | Tuna* (canned in oil and drained), salmon* (canned). | ¼ cup |
| *Cheese:* | Skim or part-skim milk cheeses, such as: | |
| | Ricotta | ¼ cup |
| | Mozzarella | 1 ounce |
| | Diet cheeses* with 56-80 calories per ounce | 1 ounce |
| *Other:* | 86 percent fat-free luncheon meat* | 1 ounce |
| | Egg (high in cholesterol, limit to 3 per week) | 1 |
| | Egg substitutes with 56-80 calories per ¼ cup | ¼ cup |
| | Tofu (2-½ x 2-¾ x 1 inches) | 4 ounces |
| | Liver, heart, kidney, sweetbreads (high in cholesterol) | 1 ounce |

## HIGH-FAT MEAT AND SUBSTITUTES

Remember, these items are high in saturated fat, cholesterol, and calories, and should be used only three times per week. One exchange is equal to any one of the following items.

| | | |
|---|---|---|
| *Beef:* | Most USDA prime cuts of beef, such as ribs, corned beef* | 1 ounce |
| *Pork:* | Spareribs, ground pork, pork sausage* (patty or link) | 1 ounce |
| *Lamb:* | Patties (ground lamb) | 1 ounce |
| *Fish:* | Any fried fish product | 1 ounce |
| *Cheese:* | All regular cheeses*, such as American, Blue, Cheddar, Monterey, Swiss | 1 ounce |
| *Other:* | Luncheon meat*, such as bologna, salami, pimento loaf | 1 ounce |
| | Sausage*, such as Polish, Italian, knockwurst, smoked | 1 ounce |
| | Bratwurst* | 1 ounce |
| | Frankfurter* (turkey or chicken) | 1 frank (10 per pound) |
| | Peanut Butter (contains unsaturated fat) | 1 tablespoon |

*Count as one High-Fat Meat plus one Fat Exchange:*

| | | |
|---|---|---|
| | Frankfurter* (beef, pork, or combination) | 1 frank (10 per pound) |

I often buy a round roast on special, have the fat trimmed off and have it ground into extra lean ground beef. It has wonderful flavor, is usually less expensive than ground meat with much higher fat content. This truly makes for very lean ground beef.

9

## LIST 3
## VEGETABLE EXCHANGES

Each vegetable serving on this list contains approximately 5 grams of carbohydrate, 2 grams of protein, and 25 calories. Vegetables contain 2 to 3 grams of dietary fiber.

Vegetables are a good source of vitamins and minerals. Fresh and frozen vegetables have more vitamins and less added salt. Rinsing canned vegetables in cool water will remove much of the salt.

Unless otherwise noted, the serving size for vegetables is:

- ½ cup of cooked vegetables or vegetable juice
- 1 cup of raw vegetables

| | | |
|---|---|---|
| Artichoke (½ medium) | Cauliflower | Rutabaga |
| | Eggplant | Sauerkraut* |
| Asparagus | Greens (collard, mustard, turnip) | Spinach, cooked |
| Beans (green, wax, Italian) | Kohlrabi | Summer squash (crookneck) |
| Bean sprouts | Leeks | Tomato (one large) |
| Beets | Mushrooms, cooked | Tomato/vegetable juice* |
| Broccoli | Okra | |
| Brussels sprouts | Onions | Turnips |
| Cabbage, cooked | Pea pods | Water chestnuts |
| Carrots | Peppers (green) | Zucchini, cooked |

Starchy vegetables such as corn, peas, and potatoes are found on the Starch/Bread List.

For free vegetables, see the Free Food List at the end of this section.

*400 milligrams or more of sodium per serving.

*3 grams or more of fiber per serving.

Rhubarb is botanically a vegetable but we treat it like a fruit.

If the stem end of carrots are discolored they are too mature. The sweet carrot taste comes from the bright orange core where the sugar is stored.

Fresh vegetables are one of our best convenience foods. They are ready in a jiffy . . . stir-fried in a jiffy or full of flavor crisp and raw.

Most green vegetables will stay crisp longest if refrigerated in plastic bags or a covered container. Vegetables that have been washed should be drained to store.

**LIST 4**

## FRUIT EXCHANGES

Each item on this list contains about 15 grams of carbohydrate, and 60 calories. Fresh, frozen, and dry fruits have about 2 grams of fiber per serving. Fruit juices contain very little dietary fiber.

The carbohydrate and calorie content for a fruit serving are based on the usual serving of the most commonly eaten fruits. Use fresh fruits, or fruits frozen or canned without sugar added. Whole fruit is more filling than fruit juice, and may be a better choice for those who are trying to lose weight. Unless otherwise noted, the serving size for fruit is:

- ½ cup of fresh fruit or fruit juice
- ¼ cup of dried fruit

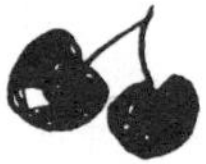

### FRESH, FROZEN, AND UNSWEETENED CANNED FRUIT

| | |
|---|---|
| Apple (raw, 2 inches across) | 1 apple |
| Applesauce (unsweetened) | ½ cup |
| Apricots (medium, raw) | 4 apricots |
| Apricots (canned) | ½ cup, or 4 halves |
| Banana (9 inches long) | ½ banana |
| Blackberries* (raw) | ¾ cup |
| Blueberries* (raw) | ¾ cup |
| Cantaloupe (cubed) | 1 cup |
| Cantaloupe (5 inches across) | ⅓ melon |
| Cherries (large, sweet, raw) | 12 cherries |
| Cheries (canned) | ½ cup |
| Figs (raw, 2 inches across) | 2 figs |
| Fruit cocktail (canned) | ½ cup |
| Grapefruit (medium) | ½ grapefruit |
| Grapefruit (segments) | ¾ cup |
| Grapes (small) | 15 grapes |
| Guava (fresh) | 1 medium |
| Guava (pulp | ½ cup |
| Honeydew melon (medium) | ⅛ melon |
| Honeydew melon (cubed) | 1 cup |
| Kiwi (large) | 1 kiwi |
| Lychees | 8 fruits |

| | |
|---|---|
| Mandarin oranges | ¾ cup |
| Mango (small) | ½ mango |
| Nectarine* (1-½ inches across) | 1 nectarine |
| Orange (2-½ inches across) | 1 orange |
| Papaya | 1 cup |
| Peach (2-¾ inches across) | 1 peach, or ¾ cup |
| Peaches (canned) | ½ cup, or 2 havles |
| Pear | ½ large, 1 small |
| Pears (canned) | ½ cup, or 2 halves |
| Persimmon (medium, native, crisp) | 2 persimmons |
| Persimmon (Japanese, bell shaped, soft) | ½ medium |
| Pineapple (raw) | ¾ cup |
| Pineapple (canned) | ⅓ cup |
| Plum (raw, 2 inches across) | 2 plums |
| Poha | ½ cup |
| Pomegranate* | ½ pomegranate |
| Raspberries* (raw) | 1 cup |
| Soursop, pulp | ½ cup |
| Strawberries* (raw, whole) | 1-¼ cup |
| Surinam | 20 cherries |
| Tangerine* (2-½ inches across) | 2 tangerines |
| Watermelon (cubes) | 1-¼ cups |

### DRIED FRUIT

| | |
|---|---|
| Apples* | 4 rings |
| Apricots* | 7 halves |
| Dates | 2-½ medium |
| Figs* | 1-½ |
| Prunes* | 3 medium |
| Raisins | 2 tablespoons |

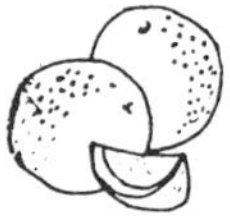

### FRUIT JUICE

| | |
|---|---|
| Apple juice/cider | ½ cup |
| Cranberry juice cocktail | ⅓ cup |
| Grapefruit juice | ½ cup |
| Grape juice | ⅓ cup |
| Orange juice | ½ cup |
| Passion fruit juice | ⅓ cup |
| Pineapple juice | ½ cup |
| Prune juice | ⅓ cup |

## LIST 5

### MILK EXCHANGES

Each serving of milk or milk products on this list contains approximately 12 grams of carbohydrate and 8 grams of protein. The amount of fat in milk is measured in percent of butterfat. The calories vary, depending on what kind of milk you choose. The list is divided into three parts based on the amount of fat and calories: skim/very low-fat milk, low-fat milk, and whole milk. One serving (1 Milk Exchange) of each of these includes:

|  | Carbohydrate (grams) | Protein (grams) | Fat (grams) | Calories |
|---|---|---|---|---|
| Skim/Very Low-Fat | 12 | 8 | trace | 90 |
| Low-Fat | 12 | 8 | 5 | 120 |
| Whole | 12 | 8 | 8 | 150 |

Milk is the body's main source of calcium, the mineral needed for growth and repair of bones. Yogurt is also a good source of calcium. Yogurt and many dry or powdered milk products have different amounts of fat. If you have questions about a particular item, read the label to find out the fat and calorie content in the product.

Milk is good to drink, but it can also be added to cereal, and used in cooking with other foods.

### SKIM AND VERY LOW-FAT MILK

1 cup skim milk
1 cup ½ percent milk
1 cup 1 percent milk
1 cup low-fat buttermilk
½ cup evaporated skim milk
⅓ cup dry nonfat milk
8-ounce carton plain nonfat yogurt

### LOW-FAT MILK

1 cup fluid 2 percent milk
8-ounce carton plain low-fat yogurt (with added nonfat milk solids)

### WHOLE MILK

The whole milk group has much more fat per serving than the skim and low-fat groups. Whole milk has more than 3-¼ percent butterfat. Try to limit your choices from the whole milk group.

1 cup whole milk
½ cup evaporated whole milk
8-ounce carton whole plain yogurt

*400 milligrams or more of sodium per serving.

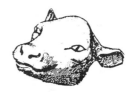

## LIST 6

# FAT EXCHANGE

Each serving on the fat list contains about 5 grams of fat and 45 calories.

The foods on the fat list contain mostly fat, although some items may also contain a small amount of protein. All fats are high in calories, and should be carefully measured. Everyone should modify fat intake by eating unsaturated fats instead of saturated fats. The sodium content of these foods varies widely. Check the label for sodium information.

## UNSATURATED FATS

| | |
|---|---|
| Avocado | ⅛ medium |
| Margarine | 1 teaspoon |
| Margarine, diet* | 1 tablespoon |
| Mayonnaise | 1 teaspoon |
| Mayonnaise, reduced-calorie* | 1 tablespoon |
| Nuts and Seeds: | |
|    Almonds, dry roasted | 6 whole |
|    Cashews, dry roasted | 1 tablespoon |
|    Pecans | 2 whole |
|    Peanuts | 20 small, 10 large |
|    Walnuts | 2 whole |
|    Other nuts | 1 tableploon |
|    Seeds, pine nuts, sunflower (without shells) | 1 tablespoon |
|    Pumpkin seeds | 2 teaspoons |
| Oil (corn, cottonseed, safflower, sesame, soybean, sunflower, olive, peanut) | 1 teaspoon |
| Olives* | 10 small, 5 large |
| Salad dressing, mayonnaise-type | 2 teaspoons |
| Salad dressing, mayonnaise-type, reduced-calorie | 1 tablespoon |
| Salad dressing (all varieties)* | 1 tablespoon |
| Salad dressing, reduced-calorie† | 2 tablespoons |

## SATURATED FATS

| | |
|---|---|
| Butter | 1 teaspoon |
| Bacon* | 1 slice |
| Chitterlings | ½ ounce |
| Coconut | |
|    Shredded | 2 tablespoons |
|    Mature meat | 1 piece (1" x 1" x ⅜") |
|    Cream, no water added | 2 tablespoons |
|    Milk (1 cup water to 1 cup cream) | 3 tablespoons |
|    Coconut, grated | 2-½ tablespoons |
| Coffee whitener, liquid | 2 tablespoons |
| Coffee whitener, powder | 4 teaspoons |
| Cream (light, coffee, table) | 2 tablespoons |
| Cream, sour | 2 tablespoons |
| Cream (heavy, whipping) | 1 tablespoon |
| Cream cheese | 1 tablespoon |
| Lard | 1 teaspoon |
| Salt pork* | ¼ ounce (¾" cube) |

*If more than one or two servings are consumed, sodium levels will equal or exceed 400 milligrams.

†400 milligrams or more of sodium per serving.

(Two tablespoons of low-calorie salad dressing is a Free Food.)

*400 milligrams or more of sodium per serving.

*3 grams or more of fiber per serving.

# FREE FOODS

A free food is any food or drink that contains 20 calories or less per serving. You can eat as much as you want of those items that have no serving size specified. You may eat two or three servings per day of those items that have a specific serving size. Be sure to spread them out through the day or they will need to be calculated into your diet.

## DRINKS

Bouillon,† or broth without fat
Bouillon, low sodium
Carbonated drinks, sugar-free
Carbonated water
Club soda
Cocoa powder, unsweetened (1 tablespoon)
Coffee/Tea
Drink mixes, sugar-free
Mineral water
Tonic water, sugar-free

## Nonstick pan spray

## Fruit

Cranberries, unsweetened (½ cup)
Rhubarb, unsweetened (½ cup)

*If more than one or two servings are consumed, sodium levels will equal or exceed 400 milligrams.

## Vegetables (raw, 1 cup)

Cabbage
Celery
Chinese cabbage*
Cucumber

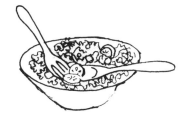

Green onion
Hot peppers
Mushrooms
Radishes
Seaweed
Zucchini*
Salad greens:
  Endive
  Escarole
  Lettuce
  Romaine
  Spinach

## Condiments

Catsup (1 tablespoon)
Horseradish
Mustard
Pickles*, dill, unsweetened
Salad dressing, low-calorie (2 tablespoons)
Taco sauce (1 tablespoon)

Seasonings can be very helpful in making food taste better. Be careful of how much sodium you use. Read the label, and choose seasonings that do not contain sodium or salt.

| | | |
|---|---|---|
| Basil (fresh) | Garlic | Paprika |
| Celery seeds | Garlic powder | Pepper |
| Cinnamon | Herbs | Pimento |
| Chili powder | Hot pepper sauce | Spices |
| Chives | Lemon | Soy sauce* (Shoyu) |
| Curry | Lemon juice | Soy sauce, low |
| Dill | Lemon pepper |   sodium |
| Flavoring extracts | Lime | Wine, used in |
|   (vanilla, lemon, | Lime juice |   cooking (¼ cup) |
|   almond, walnut, | Mint | Worcestershire sauce |
|   peppermint, butter, | Onion powder | |
|   and the like) | Oregano | |

# BREAKFAST AND BREADS

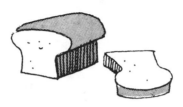

## SWEET OATMEAL

Serves 2
1 Serving = 130 Calories
1/2 Fruit Exchange
1-1/4 Bread/Starch Exchanges

C = 26.5  P = 4  F = Trace

1/2 cup apple juice
1 cup water
1/4 teaspoon cinnamon
1/4 teaspoon nutmeg
2/3 cup old fashioned rolled oats

Combine apple juice, water, cinnamon and nutmeg in sauce pan that can be covered on high heat. Bring to a boil and stir in oats. Turn heat down to simmer and cook 8 to 10 minutes, stirring three times. Cover pan, remove from heat and let rest for 2-3 minutes before serving.

# ENGLISH MUFFIN BREAD

Makes 16 slices
Each slice = 100 Calories
1-¼ Bread Exchange
Milk Exchange negligible

C = 19  P = 4  F = Trace

3 cups flour, divided
1 envelope (1 tablespoon) dry yeast
1 teaspoon salt
⅛ teaspoon baking soda
1 cup skim milk
¼ cup water
Corn meal (about 1 tablespoon)

Combine 1-½ cups of the flour, the yeast, salt and baking soda in a large bowl. In a small saucepan, heat the milk and water until very warm (120 to 130 degrees). Add the liquids to the dry mixture and beat well. Stir in the remaining flour to make a stiff batter. Grease an 8-½ by 4-½ by 2-½ inch loaf pan; sprinkle with cornmeal. Place the batter in the pan and sprinkle the top lightly with cornmeal. Cover and let rise in a warm place for about 1 hour. Bake in 400-degree oven for 25 to 30 minutes, until done and lightly brown. Remove from the pan and cool upright on a baking rack.

Note:  Batter bread of this type may also be baked in a glass or microwave-proof plastic loaf pan in a microwave oven. It should be baked for 6-½ minutes. It will not brown, but since this type of bread is usually toasted, anyway, the color is not as important as with some other breads.
*  Great Toasted!
*  Nice, chewy fat free bread — so enjoy your fat exchanges as melted butter drips in all the little nooks and crannies.

# HOMEMADE RAISIN BREAD

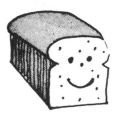

Makes 2 loaves
1 Slice = 125 Calories
1 Bread Exchange
Skim Milk Negligible
Fruit Negligible
1 Fat Exchange

C = 15  P = 3  F = 5

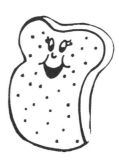

2 bread pans
4 cups unsifted flour
1 package active dry yeast
½ cup water
½ cup skim milk
½ cup butter or margarine (no shortening, please)
1 teaspoon salt
½ cup raisins
2 eggs
¼ cup chopped nuts

Mix 2 cups of the flour with the yeast in a large mixing bowl and set aside. In a medium saucepan mix water, milk, butter and salt and heat gently over low heat just until butter melts. Take off the burner and let cool for 5 minutes. Add the flour and yeast in a large bowl. Mix well. Add the rest of the flour, raisins, eggs and nuts. Stir hard as dough will be stiff. Knead on a floured board (can be counter top or table) until dough is smooth and raisins are well mixed about. Divide the dough in half and shape into loaf. Place dough in bread pan that has been lightly greased with shortening. Let rise in warm

*still more of the . . .* **HOMEMADE RAISIN BREAD**

place (about 85 degrees) until nearly double in size. (Takes between an hour and an hour and a half). Bake at 375 degrees about 35 minutes until top sounds hollow when tapped and cake tester comes out clean.

* This is also fun to bake in 2 1-pound coffee cans. Just use the cans in place of the bread pans. It will rise to about 1 inch from the top when it's ready to bake. Fun for a party or picnics.
* Raisin bread spread with cream type cheese is delicious served with a fruit or vegetable salad meal.

## QUICK DONUTS

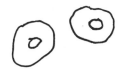

10 Servings
1 Serving = 148 Calories
1 Bread Exchange
1-½ Fat Exchange

C = 15  P = 3  F = 7.5

1 tube refrigerator biscuits
1 cup oil

Heat oil in small sauce pan with high sides. Flatten out biscuits and poke a hole in the middle with your finger. When oil begins to lightly smoke add biscuits one at a time. With tongs turn biscuits over when brown and fluffy. Remove and place on paper towel to cool. Super dipped in strawberry topping.

## APPLE SWIRL BREAD

Makes 20 Slices
1 Bread Exchange
2/5 Fruit Exchange
1/4 Fat Exchange
115 Calories

C = 19.5   P = 3   F = 1.5

1 loaf frozen bread dough
2 tablespoons butter or margarine, room temperature
½ cup apple juice concentrate, room temperature
2 medium apples, peeled and chopped
½ teaspoon cinnamon

Let bread dough defrost until soft and pliable and starting to rise. With hands flatten into a rectangle about 8" x 14". Spread dough with butter or margarine – reserving 1 teaspoon to grease the bread pan. Mix chopped apples with 2-3 tablespoons apple juice concentrate and cinnamon. Put apple mixture on buttered dough. Roll dough jelly roll style from the 8" end. Pour remaining concentrate in buttered pan. Place roll in pan. Let rise until double in size. Preheat oven to 350 degrees. Bake about 30 minutes, until brown and hollow sounding when tapped on top. Cool in pan 10 minutes. Remove from pan carefully — syrup in bottom will be hot! Spoon syrup over top. Enjoy!

*   This is always a diabetic class favorite!

# RAISIN-APPLE STICKY BUNS
## * Everybody's favorite!

Makes 20 Rolls
1 Roll = (without nuts)
1 Bread Exchange
½ Fruit Exchange
¼ Fat Exchange
125 Calories

C = 22.5  P = 3  F = 1.2

(with nuts) 1 Roll Equals
1 Bread Exchange
½ Fat Exchange
½ Fruit Exchange
135 Calories

C = 22.5  P = 3  F = 2.5

1 loaf frozen bread dough
2 tablespoons butter or margarine, room temperature
½ cup apple juice concentrate, room temperature
6 tablespoons raisins (golden are pretty)
2 medium apples, peeled and chopped
½ teaspoon cinnamon
½ cup chopped walnuts — or pecans (if desired)

Remove dough from plastic package. Let dough defrost until soft, pliable and starting to rise. Divide in half. Flatten each half into rectangles about ⅓ inch thick. Spread each half with half of butter (reserve a bit of the butter — to lightly grease a 9 x 13 baking dish). In a small bowl, mix chopped apple, cinnamon, 4 tablespoons chopped nuts, raisins and 3 tablespoons apple juice concentrate. Pour remaining concentrate in lightly buttered pan. Sprinkle remaining nuts over apple juice concentrate in pan. Spread ½ apple filling mix over each buttered rectangle. Roll jelly roll style from long side. Cut each roll into 10 slices and place on nut/concentrate mix in pan. Cover with clean towel and let rise until doubled. Preheat oven to 350 degrees. Bake sticky buns 20-25 minutes until golden brown and hollow sounding when tapped. Let cool in pan 8-10 minutes. Invert on large serving platter and serve warm.
* May be baked in 2 - 8 inch round cake pans.    * Best first day!
* Invert pan while still quite warm so sticky syrup drips over rolls.

# HOMEMADE WHOLE WHEAT BRAN BREAD

### (Delicious — quick and no need to knead!)

2-¾ cups whole wheat flour
½ cup dry milk powder
1 envelope quick rising active dry yeast
¼ cup apple juice concentrate
1-¼ cups warm water (110 – 115 degrees farenheit)
1-½ cups 100% Bran cereal
1 egg
3 tablespoons vegetable oil

Makes 20 slices
1 Slice Equals
1 Starch/Bread Exchange
Milk Negligible
Fruit Negligible
¼ Fat Exchange
90 Calories
C = 15   P = 3   F = 1.5

Lighly grease one 9" x 5" bread pan and set aside. If desired sprinkle 1 teaspoon Bran cereal in bottom of greased pan for an interesting texture. In a large mixing bowl combine the yeast, warm water and apple juice concentrate and stir until yeast is dissolved. Add the 100% Bran cereal and let stand 2 minutes so the cereal can soften. Beat in the egg and the oil. Add the dry milk powder and one cup of whole wheat flour and beat until smooth. Add the remaining flour and beat until all flour is blended in. Shape loaf and place in bread pan. Cover with a towel and let rise in a warm place until bread reaches top of loaf pan — usually about 40-45 minutes. Top will be nicely brown and loaf will sound hollow when tapped on top. Cool in the pan for 5 minutes and then finish cooling out of the pan on a wire rack.

*   For best results the water, apple juice concentrate mix should be about 110-115 degrees farenheit to activate the yeast. Too hot — will destroy the yeast — too cool will not activate it properly.

*   A wooden spoon works best to beat this bread.

*   One packet of the quick rising yeast equals one packet active dry yeast and may be interchanged. Rising time is increased to about an hour with regular active dry yeast.

*   This is a nice light, moist wheat bread that is excellent for sandwiches, toast and adds good fiber.

*   Homemade bread — in almost less time than a trip to the bakery!

21

# DATE MYSTERY BREAD

(A hearty batter bread that disappears!)

Makes 1 Loaf
18 ½" Thick Slices
1 Slice Equals
⅔ Bread Exchange
¾ Fruit Exchange
½ Fat Exchange
Medium Fat Meat Negligible
125 Calories

C = 22   P = 3   F = 2.5

1 cup unsugared dates, chopped
¾ cup raisins
1-½ cups boiling water
2 cups whole wheat flour (regular not bread flour)
1 teaspoon baking soda
1 teaspoon baking powder
1 large egg
1 teaspoon vanilla
½ cup chopped walnuts (not too fine)

Preheat oven to 350 degrees. Grease lightly a 9 x 5 x 3 inch bread pan. In a small bowl combine dates, raisins and boiling water. Set aside. In a large mixing bowl mix together flour, baking soda & baking powder. Beat egg and vanilla into date mixture. Combine date mixture with dry ingredients in bowl and mix well. Spread batter in prepared bread pan. Bake 45-50 minutes until a toothpick inserted in the center comes out clean. Let rest in pan 10-15 minutes and move to wine rack. Wrap well to stow.

* I usually but an 8 ounce package of whole dates and cut them into bits with my "cooking" scissors. These usually are more moist.

* This bread develops flavor as it stands and is best the second day.

* Serve plain or spread lightly with cream cheese.

# CORNMEAL BISCUITS

Makes 10 Biscuits
1 Biscuit Equals
1 Starch/Bread Exchange
1 Fat Exchange
125 Calories

C = 15   P = 3   F = 5

⅓ cup shortening
1-¼ cup flour
½ cup cornmeal
2-½ teaspoons baking powder
¼ teaspoon salt
¾ cup very low fat milk
1 tablespoon additional cornmeal

Preheat oven to 450 degrees.  Combine flour, ½ cup cornmeal, baking powder and salt in small mixing bowl.  Add shortening and with a knife cut shortening into dry mix until the pieces are the size of fine crumbs. Stir in milk so the dough forms a ball. Turn ball out onto a lightly floured surface and knead lightly 12 to 15 times.  Roll or pat dough into a circle ½ inch thick.  Cut into 2" rounds with biscuit cutter or drinking glass.  Sprinkle ungreased cookie sheet with 2 teaspoons cornmeal.  Place biscuits next to each other on cookie sheet. Sprinkle with 1 teaspoon cornmeal.  Bake 10 minutes or until light brown.  Remove from cookie sheet.

*   If the sides touch when biscuits bake they will be soft. Baked apart biscuits will be crispy.

## CHEESE-ONION BISCUITS

Knead in ½ cup grated sharp cheddar cheese and ¼ cup finely chopped green onions into cornmeal biscuits above.  Bake 12 to 15 minutes until light brown. Add 23 calories

# RAISIN-APPLESAUCE MUFFINS

1 large egg
2 tablespoons vegetable oil
1-½ cups unsweetened applesauce
2 cups flour
½ teaspoon baking soda
2 teaspoons baking powder
1 teaspoon cinnamon
¾ cup raisins

Makes 12
1 Muffin Equals
1 Bread Exchange
¾ Fruit Exchange
½ Fat Exchange
Medium Fat Meat Negligible
153 Calories
C = 27   P = 3.5   F = 3

Preheat oven to 375 degrees.  Line muffin tin with muffin papers and set aside.

Mix raisins and ¼ cup applesauce.  Beat together egg, oil, and 1-¼ cups applesauce.  Add flour, baking soda, baking powder, and cinnamon.  Mix until moistened.  Stir in raisin-applesauce mix.  Spoon batter into muffin pans.  Bake for 20 to 25 minutes or until firm to the touch and browned.  Cool on wire racks.  Serve warm.

# RAISIN-NUT APPLESAUCE MUFFINS

Makes 12
1 Muffin Equals
1 Bread Exchange
¾ Fruit Exchange
¾ Medium Fat Meat Exchange
170 Calories

C = 27   P = 3.5   F = 4

Stir ¼ cup chopped walnuts to Raisin-Applesauce muffins when adding raisins.

*   Raisin Nut Muffins are much like an applesauce cake.  Frost with french pastry icing for delicious cupcakes.

# ZUCCHINI BREAD

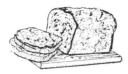

Serves 16
1 Slice Equals
⅔ Bread Exchange
1-¼ Fat Exchange
⅓ Fruit Exchange
Vegetable negligible
Milk negligible
Medium Fat Meat negligible
136 Calories

$C = 15.25$   $P = 2.75$   $F = 6.5$

½ cup zucchini, grated and patted dry
1-½ cups flour
¼ cup non fat dry milk powder
1 teaspoon baking soda
¼ teaspoon salt
⅓ cup oil
1 egg
1 8-¾ ounce can crushed pineapple in juice
½ cup raisins
½ cup chopped nuts

Preheat oven to 350 degrees. Lightly grease a 9" x 5" x 3" loaf pan. Grate zucchini, squeeze out excess moisture and pat dry with paper toweling. Firmly pack ½ cup measuring cup. Mix together flour, dry milk powder, baking soda and salt. Set aside. In blender container puree pineapple with juice. Add oil and egg and blend. Add liquid ingredients to dry mixture. Mix well. Stir in zucchini, nuts and raisins. Pour batter into prepared pan. Bake 60-70 minutes — until nicely browned and cake tester comes out clean. Cool on wire rack before cutting.

* Sometimes I use half white — half whole wheat flour.

* If you object to raisins in zucchini bread — puree raisins with pineapple. They provide much sweetness to the zucchini bread.

# EASY DATE POCKETS

Makes 10
1 Serving Equals
1 Bread Exchange
¼ Fruit Exchange
Fat Exchange negligible
95 Calories

$C = 18.75$  $P = 3$  $F = $ negligible

1 can buttermilk refrigerator biscuits (the kind from the grocery store deli case)
10 teaspoons date butter (page 56  )
1 teaspoon melted butter

Check can directions and preheat oven to specified temperature.  Separate biscuits and flatten with palms of hands.  Place 1 teaspoon date spread on one half of biscuit.  Fold other half over filled side and press edges shut with tines of a fork. Brush with melted butter and bake on ungreased baking sheet according to directions on the biscuit can.

# EASY DATE NUT POCKETS

Makes 10
1 Bread Exchange
⅓ Fat Exchange
¼ Fruit Exchange
110 Calories

$C = 19$   $P = 3$   $F = 1.66$

Add two tablespoons chopped nuts to date filling.  Follow directions for Easy Date Pockets.

## QUICK DATE NUT PINWHEELS
### * Good breakfast or dinner rolls

Use all ingredients for Easy Date Nut Pockets above.

Place biscuits in two rows of 5 biscuits touching on non-stick surface.  Flatten with rolling pin into a 10 x 6 inch rectangle. Spread with filling. Roll jelly roll style to form a 10" long roll.  Cut in 1 inch slices and place in 8" cake pan.  Bake as directed on biscuit can.

Values same as for Easy Date Nut Pockets.

# APPLESAUCE PANCAKES

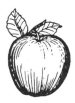

4 Servings
1 Serving =
1-½ Bread Exchanges
1-½ Fat Exchanges
¼ Fruit Exchange
¼ Skim Milk Exchange
¼ Lean Meat Exchange
245 Calories

C = 30.75  P = 8.5  F = 9

1 cup flour
¼ teaspoon salt
2 teaspoons baking powder
1 egg
1 cup skim milk
2 tablespoons vegetable oil
½ cup applesauce

Measure all ingredients and put in mixing bowl. Mix all ingredients until smooth. Cook on hot teflon griddle until bubbles form on one side. With a pancake turner carefully turn and brown on the other side.

These are special when topped with extra applesauce and sprinkled lightly with cinnamon.

# QUICK ORANGE PANCAKES

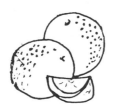

Serves 4
1 Serving Equals
1-½ Bread Exchange
½ Fat Exchange
¼ Skim Milk Exchange
½ Fruit Exchange
243 Calories

C = 40.5  P = 8.25  F = 4

1 cup pancake mix
1 egg, beaten slightly
1 cup skim milk
¼ cup orange juice concentrate, thawed
½ teaspoon grated orange peel, if desired

Combine egg, milk and orange juice concentrate in small bowl. Stir in pancake flour and beat until most lumps disappear. Add orange peel, if desired. Cook on lightly greased or non-stick griddle until bubbles form. Turn with spatula and brown on other side. Serve warm.

Good with a fruit topping or syrup.

# GERMAN PANCAKE

Serves 2
1 Serving Equals
¼ Skim Milk Exchange
1-½ Bread Exchange
1 Medium Fat Meat Exchange
1-½ Fat Exchange
290 Calories

C = 27  P = 14  F = 12.5

½ cup skim milk
½ cup flour
2 eggs
1 tablespoon melted butter
little salt, cinnamon or nutmeg (3 shakes)

Beat together by hand first three ingredients.  Melt butter in ovenproof frying pan.
Pour all ingredients into frying pan.  Sprinkle with spice.  Bake at 425 degrees for
12-15 minutes.

# FRUIT GOODIES

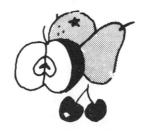

## SUNSHINE GELATIN

My daughter Carrie's favorite

Serves 6
1 Serving Equals
1/6 Vegetable Exchange
2/3 Fruit Exchange
45 Calories

$C = 11 \quad P = .33 \quad F = 0$

¾ cup orange juice
1 8-¾ ounce can crushed pineapple in pineapple juice
1 envelope unflavored gelatin
1 cup grated carrot

Place gelatin in ¼ cup orange juice to soften. Bring remaining orange juice to a boil. Mix in juice/gelatin and stir until dissolved. Add pineapple with juice and grated carrot. Stir well. Pour into mold and refrigerate until firm.

# FROZEN FRUIT CUPS

Serves 8
1 Serving Equals
⅛ Milk Exchange
½ Fat Exchange
½ Fruit Exchange
63 Calories

C = 9  P = 1  F = 2.5

1 (8 ounce) carton plain non-fat yogurt
½ cup sour cream
1-½ cups raspberries
1 (9 inch) banana, sliced
1 (8 ounce) can mandarin oranges, canned in fruit juice

Drain mandarin oranges and set aside. In a medium sized bowl mash ½ cup raspberries. Stir yogurt and sour cream into mashed berries. Gently fold in remaining berries, banana slices and drained oranges. Pour into a 4 quart mold or 8 individual molds (I like to use muffin tins lined with little paper muffin cups.) and freeze until firm. To serve unmold and let rest at room temperature about 15 minutes before eating.

*   Pretty garnished with a raspberry or orange slice.

# FROZEN YOGURT POPS

Makes 8 Pops
1 Pop Equals
¼ Milk Exchange
⅔ Fruit Exchange
60 Calories

C = 13  P = 2  F = 0

2 8 ounce cartons plain yogurt
6 ounce frozen fruit concentrate

Slush concentrate in blender. Add yogurt and blend until smooth. Pour into 3 ounce paper cups and place in freezer. When partially set insert sticks. Freeze firmly. Enjoy!

*   Grape is a favorite . . . purple and sweet!

# BAKED BANANA

Serves 4
1 Serving Equals
1 Fruit Exchange
¾ Fat Exchange
90 Calories

C = 15  P = 0  F = 3.75

2 9 inch bananas
2 teaspoons butter or margarine
2 tablespoons shredded coconut
dash of cinnamon
*few drops of lemon juice (if desired)

Preheat oven to 375 degrees. Cut bananas in half lengthwise. Dribble cut side with lemon juice to prevent darkening if desired. Melt butter and dribble evenly over banana halves. Sprinkle lightly with cinnamon and sprinkle with coconut. Bake 10-12 minutes until warm and slightly soft.

* This makes a nice warm breakfast fruit or light simple dessert that can be baked at the last minute while the rest of the meal cooks.

* If I'm in a hurry I slice the bananas into circles, melt the butter and mix with cinnamon and coconut and stir into bananas. Bake 8-10 minutes. Serve in little bowls or on french toast.

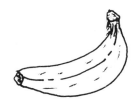

# APPLES 'n APRICOTS

Serves 2
1 Serving Equals
2 Fruit Exchanges
120 Calories

C = 30  P = 0  F = 0

AS A TOPPING
Serves 4
1 Serving Equals
1 Fruit Exchange
60 Calories

C = 15  P = 0  F = 0

8 apricot halves, canned in juice or water
1 small apple, cored and diced
½ cup orange juice
1 cinnamon stick
2-3 whole cloves

Drain apricots and combine with diced apple (peel adds color but may be removed if you prefer), orange juice, cinnamon stick and cloves in small sauce pan. Cook over medium heat 2-3 minutes (if you like a bit of crunch) or simmer 8-10 minutes for soft fruit. Remove cinnamon stick and cloves and enjoy!

* Great breakfast fruit on a cold morning!
* Good topping for waffles, french toast or pancakes.
* Serve leftovers cold for dessert topped with a dollop of whipped cream.

# APPLESAUCE

4 medium peeled, sliced apples
¼ cup apple juice concentrate
½ cup water
cinnamon or nutmeg to taste

Serves 6
1 Serving Equals
1 Fruit Exchange
60 Calories

C = 15   P = 0   F = 0

Combine all ingredients in saucepan.  Simmer covered until apples are tender – about 15-20 minutes.  Stir to mix well and break up slices.  May seive if desired.  Delicious warm or cold.  *If apples are very juicy, you may want to add only ¼ cup water.

* Quick trick – If you're in a hurry unpeeled apples may be used.  Simply cook until tender and strain or seive apples.  Sauce will be fine textured.  Season after straining.

* Apple juice may be substituted for the concentrate and water, however, you do not have the control of the amount of liquid concentrate in the sweetener.

# RAISIN BAKED APPLES

4 medium apples
¼ cup raisins
⅔ cup apple juice
cinnamon, nutmeg or apple pie spice (optional)

Serves 4
1 Serving Equals
2 Fruit Exchanges
120 Calories

C = 30   P = 0   F = 0

Preheat oven to 375 degrees.  Wash and core apples.  Peel a collar off the top of each apple and if apple won't sit up take a small slice from the bottom.  Place in baking dish. Fill each apple center with one tablespoon raisins.  Pour juice over apples and sprinkle lightly with spice, if desired.  Bake 40-45 minutes until firm, soft, basting frequently. Serve warm or chilled.

Super dessert with a dollop of whipped cream.

# FRUIT YOGURT

Serves 2
1 Serving Equals
½ Milk Exchange
½ Fruit Exchange
75 Calories

C = 13.5  P = 4  F = 0

1 8 ounce carton plain low-fat yogurt
¾ cup blueberries, blackberries, peaches or pineapple

Wash and drain fresh berries (or drain frozen berries).  Squish one half of fruit with potato masher and stir into yogurt.  Add the remaining whole berries and mix gently — divide into two dishes and enjoy!  Great for breakfast or dessert.

*   Don't use the mixer as yogurt will get a bit watery if over mixed.

Serves 2
1 Serving = 90 Calories
½ Milk Exchange
¾ Fruit Exchange

C = 18  P = 4  F = Trace

A BIT OUT OF THE ORDINARY . . . stir ½ cup grape halves in low-fat yogurt and sprinkle with a dash of nutmeg.  Cool and crunchy.

# SWEET FRUIT SOUP

Serves 8
1 Serving Equals
1-¼ Fruit Exchanges
¼ Bread Exchange
95 Calories

C = 22  P = 1  F = trace

1 8 ounce package mixed dried fruit (apples, pears, prunes, apricots w/o pits)
½ cup light or golden raisins
1-½ cups water
¼ cup tapioca
1 cup red or light grape juice
1 stick cinnamon

In sauce pan combine tapioca and water over medium heat and bring to boil. Cut the dried fruit in bite size pieces. Add raisins, dried fruit pieces and cinnamon stick. Simmer until fruit is tender and thickened (30-40 minutes). Stir in grape juice. Remove cinnamon stick and enjoy!

Good hot or cold. Refrigerate any leftovers.

* Great first course at brunch — festive served in a stemmed glass.
* Nice for dessert with a dollop of whipped cream.
* Thickens a bit when left over and may be enjoyed heated and used as a topping for waffles or pancakes.

# SPICY MANDARIN ORANGES

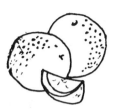

Serves 6
1 Serving Equals
1 Fruit Exchange
Bread negligible
65 Calories
C = 16  P = .5  F = 0
With 1 tablespoon whipped cream
add ½ fat exchange
23 calories
2.5 gm fat

1 11 oz. can unsweetened mandarin oranges in fruit juice
1-½ cups orange juice
4 teaspoons minute tapioca
¼ teaspoon ground ginger or cinnamon

Drain juice from mandarin oranges and mix with orange juice and tapioca in sauce pan. Over low heat, cook stirring occasionally until mixture boils. Remove from heat and stir in spice. Add drained oranges stirring gently to mix but not breaking fruit sections. Cool. Serve lukewarm or chilled.

* Excellent topped with a dollop of whipped cream.
* A brunch treat served warm on a waffle and sprinkled with a pinch of shredded coconut.
* Served cold in individual dishes for dessert with whipped cream it's fruit pudding.

# APRICOT WHIP

Serves 4
1 Serving Equals
1 Fruit Exchange
Meat Exchange negligible
65 Calories

$C = 15$   $P = 1$   $F = $ trace

16 apricot halves canned in juice or water
1 envelope unflavored gelatin
¼ teaspoon almond extract
¼ cup boiling water
2 egg whites

Place apricot halves in blender container and blend until smooth. Dissolve gelatin in boiling water and stir into apricot mix with almond extract. Refrigerate until slightly thickened. Beat egg whites until stiff (but not dry) and fold into apricot mix. Spoon into serving dishes and refrigerate.

* Pretty served in a stemmed (wine type) glass garnished with a fresh fruit bit or lemon twist.

## PEAR CLOWNS
### What child can resist a dessert that smiles?

Makes 2
1 Serving Equals
½ Fruit Exchange
Vegetable negligible
30 Calories

1 peeled fresh or canned pear, halved
4 raisins
fresh carrot-grated or in curls
1 cherry, sliced

$C = 7.5$  $P = 0$  $F = 0$

Place pear cut side down on small plate. Use raisins for eyes and cherry pieces for nose and mouth. Garnish with carrot hair. A real treat for little ones.

*   A few carrot shreds make a good mustache for "boy" clowns.

## GRANNY PEARS

1 peeled fresh or canned pear, halved
½ cup cottage cheese
4 raisins
1 cherry, sliced
2 lettuce leaves (curly is best – red or green)

Makes 2
1 Serving Equals
½ Fruit Exchange
1 Lean Meat Exchange
85 Calories

$C = 7.5$  $P = 7$  $F = 3$

Follow directions for Pear Clowns except place pear half near stem end on lettuce leaf for bonnet and make cottage cheese hair.

# BAKED PEAR ON THE HALF SHELL

Serves 4
1 Serving Equals
1-½ Fruit Exchange
¼ Fat Exchange
102 Calories

$C = 22.5 \quad P = 0 \quad F = 1.25$

2 large fresh baking pears (Bosc are best)
3 tablespoons apple pear concentrate
5 tablespoons boiling water
½ teaspoon cinnamon
Raisin or date filling (below)

Raisin Filling
Combine ¼ cup raisins and 2 tablespoons chopped walnuts.

Date Filling
Combine 4 chopped dates, 2 tablespoons chopped nuts and ½ teaspoon grated orange peel (optional).

Preheat oven to 350 degrees. Halve and core pear. Fill each center with one fourth of the raisin or date filling and place in a 8 inch square baking dish. Combine boiling water, concentrate and cinnamon and pour over pears. Bake 35-40 minutes, until tender, basting frequently with syrup.

* Good warm or cold.

## BAKED APPLES ON THE HALF SHELL

Substitute large apples for pears and apple juice concentrate for apple pear concentrate. Values are the same as if using pears.

## "ADULT" BAKED PEARS

4 medium fresh pears
1 cup red grape juice
½ cup dry white wine
½ teaspoon cinnamon
1 tablespoon cornstarch
½ cup cold water

Serves 8
1 Serving =
1-¼ Fruit Exchanges
Lean Meat negligible
* alcohol evaporates from wine
75 Calories

C = 19  P = 0  F = 0

Halve and core pears and place cut side up in baking dish. (If skins are tender they may be left on — otherwise peal pears) Mix grape juice, wine and cinnamon. Pour over pears. Cover and bake at 350 degrees until tender — about 30 minutes. Mix cornstarch and water in small sauce pan. Add liquid from pear and cook until thickened. Pour sauce over pears. Good warm or cold.

## GINGER PEARS

2 small pears
1 half inch piece ginger root
1 cup pineapple juice, unsweetened

Serves 4
One Serving Equals
1 Fruit Exchange
60 Calories

C = 15  P = 0  F = 0

Simmer pineapple juice with ginger root 10 minutes. Peel pears. Cut in half and remove cores. Place pears in juice and simmer 10 minutes. Pears will be warm through and tender.

* Delicious plain or with a dollop of whipped cream or yogurt.

# INDIVIDUAL APPLESAUCE SOUFFLE

2 cups unsweetened applesauce
2 tablespoons frozen apple juice concentrate
1 teaspoon grated orange peel, if desired
¼ teaspoon cinnamon or nutmeg
4 egg whites

Serves 5
1 Serving = Equals
1 Fruit Exchange
¼ Lean Meat Exchange
75 Calories
C = 15  P = 2  F = 1

In a small bowl mix applesauce, apple juice concentrate, orange peel, and spice. Set aside. Beat egg whites until stiff and glossy. Fold applesauce mix into egg whites gently. Spoon immediately into custard or individual ramkins. Bake at 350 degrees until lightly browned — 15 to 20 minutes. Serve immediately — warm.

\* This recipe is easily cut in half to make only 3 servings.

# BAKED APPLES

Serves 4
1 Serving Equals
1-½ Fruit Exchanges
90 Calories

C = 22.5  P = 0  F = 0

4 medium apples
⅔ cup apple juice
½ teaspoon cinnamon or apple pie spice

Preheat oven to 375 degrees. Wash and core apples. Peel a collar off the top of each apple (if apple won't sit up — take a small slice from the bottom). Place in baking dish. Mix apple juice and spice. Pour over apples. Bake 40-45 minutes until firm, soft, basting frequently. Serve warm or chilled spooning over apples.

## FRUIT GEL

Berry Gel Serves 4
Grape Gel serves 6
Apple Gel serves 4
Orange Gel serves 4
Pineapple Gel serves 4
1 Serving Equals
1 Fruit Exchange
60 Calories

$C = 15 \quad P = 0 \quad F = 0$

Make your own gelatin by heating one cup of fruit juice and one envelope unflavored gelatin. When mixture boils add one cup of cold juice. This has super flavor and servings are equal to the amount of juice allowed for the fruit exchange of the type of juice used. Grape and apple are my favorites. For dessert top with whipped cream.

## FRUITY WHIP

Berry Whip serves 8
Apple Whip serves 8
Grape Whip serves 12
1 Serving Equals
½ Fruit Exchange
30 Calories

$C = 7.5 \quad P = 0 \quad F = 0$

Prepare fruit gel in a large mixing bowl. Chill stirring occasionally until almost set. (Will be very thick and get lumpy when stirred.) Remove from refrigerator and beat at high speed with mixer until foamy and about triple in volume. Pour into a large mold or individual serving dishes and chill until set. A nice light sweet dessert with few calories. Berry, apple and grape are the sweetest dessert whipped.

## JELLED FRUIT WHIP PARFAITS

Servings same as Fruit Gel
1 Serving Equals
1 Fruit Exchange
60 Calories

$C = 15 \quad P = 0 \quad F = 0$

Make basic fruit gel. Pour half mixture into stem type dessert or parfait glasses. Refrigerate individual glasses and remaining gelatin/juice mix. When remaining gelatin/juice mix gets syrupy beat with mixer to foam. Spoon foam in equal amounts on gelatin in individual dishes. Refrigerate until firm.

* Nice cool light dessert.
* Really extends fruit exchanges!

## BERRY GELATIN DESSERT

1 cup red grape juice or fruit/berry juice
1 cup boiling water
1 envelope unflavored gelatin
1-¼ cup sliced strawberries or
   1 cup fresh raspberries
¼ cup (4 tablespoons) whipped cream

Serves 4
1 Serving Equals
1 Fruit Exchange
½ Fat Exchange
Lean Meat negligible
85 Calories

$C = 15 \quad P = 0 \quad F = 2.5$

Combine gelatin and juice in small bowl stirring to dissolve gelatin. Add boiling water and stir to mix. Divide berries equally into four dessert dishes. Pour gelatin mix over top. Chill until set. Top with whipped cream – 1 tablespoon per serving.

# FRUITY DESSERT TOPPING

Makes 1-½ cups
Serves 8
1 Serving Equals
1 Fat Exchange
⅛ Fruit Exchange
55 Calories

½ cups whipping cream (1 cup whipped)
½ cup crushed pineapple canned in juice

Drain pineapple while whipping cream. Blot drained pineapple on paper towels. Fold pineapple in whipped cream. Cover and chill.
* Too much pineapple juice will cause the topping to be runny.
* Delicious on fresh, or frozen or canned fruit.
* For an elegant touch anytime, place fruit in a stemmed glass and top with fruity dessert topping!

# FRUIT PARFAIT

Serves 1
1 Serving Equals
1-⅛ Fruit Exchange
1 Fat Exchange
115 Calories

C = 17   P = 0   F = 5

3 tablespoons fruity dessert topping
Choice of one fruit:
Fresh ½ cup apricots, banana, kiwi or mango
¾ cup blackberries, blueberries, peaches, pears, pineapple
1 cup cantelope, papaya, honeydew melon, raspberries or sliced strawberries
Canned: ½ cup peaches, pears, apricots, cherries or fruit cocktail canned in fruit juice.
⅓ cup pineapple, canned in juice

Wash and drain fruit, if fresh, dicing fruit into bite size pieces. (Drain if using juice packed, canned fruit). Place one tablespoon fruity dessert topping in bottom of parfait glass. Layer with one half fruit, another tablespoon topping, remaining half of fruit and remaining topping.

# FROZEN BANANA TREATS

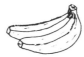

Serves 4
1 Serving Equals
1 Fruit Exchange
⅛ Bread Exchange
70 Calories

$C = 17$   $P = .5$   $F = 0$

¼ cup bran cereal (like Bran Buds, Flakes, All Bran)
1-½ tablespoons pineapple juice concentrate
2 8-½ inch bananas
4 wooden popsicle sticks or short skewers

Peel bananas and cut in half. Insert a stick in the cut end of each half. Roll each banana in the concentrate and then in cereal to coat. Freeze on flat surface uncovered until firm. When frozen wrap or drop into plastic bags and store in freezer.

* Children like the bananas rock hard — adults enjoy them most if they have been out of the freezer a few minutes before munching.

**GRAPE TREAT . . .** Frozen seedless grapes are wonderful! They are cool, refreshing and a sweet treat. Simply wash, allow to dry and pop in the freezer. Red Flame are our favorites. These are a great "finger" snack. Remember only 15 grapes equals one fruit.

# MINT FRUIT CUP

Serves 4
1 Serving Equals
1 Fruit Exchange
60 Calories

$C = 15$  $P = 0$  $F = 0$

½ cup pineapple juice (fresh or canned)
5 fresh mint leaves, chopped
1-½ cups fresh pineapple chunks
1-¼ cups fresh strawberries, halved

Combine pineapple juice and mint leaves in small sauce pan. Simmer 5 minutes over low heat. Remove from heat and let cool 15 minutes. Pour over pineapple chunks and refrigerate 1 to 2 hours to blend flavors. Before serving stir in strawberries, mixing only to coat. Enjoy!

* Cool and refreshing – makes a nice appetizer or light dessert.

* Pretty garnished with mint leaves on the side.

# RASPBERRIES WITH MINT

Serves 4
1 Serving Equals
½ Fruit Exchange
30 Calories

$C = 7.5$  $P = 0$  $F = 0$

2 cups fresh raspberries
1 tablespoon fresh mint, chopped

Wash and drain raspberries. Sprinkle with mint and fold gently to mix well. Cover tightly and refrigerate about 4 hours for flavors to blend.

* Light, unusual blend of flavors.

# JAMS, JELLIES, TOPPINGS AND SPREADS

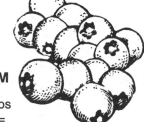

### NATURAL BLUEBERRY PEAR JAM

Makes 1-½ Cups
1 Tablespoon =
1/5 Fruit Exchange
12 Calories
C = 3  P = 0  F = 0

1 cup blueberries, washed — any stems removed
2 tablespoons water
1 cup fresh pears, peeled, cored and cubed (½ inch)
¼ cup apple juice concentrate

In medium sauce pan combine blueberries and water. Cook covered over low heat for 15 minutes, stirring every 5 minutes. Add the pears and apple juice concentrate stirring to mix. Cook an additional 15 minutes, uncovered, over medium-low heat until pears and juices reduce and jam thickens. Cool to room temperature and enjoy!

* Bartlett pears have a wonderful mellow flavor and hold their shape.

* This is delicious on hot baking powder biscuits and toast.

* Refrigerate jam to store.

49

# BLUEBERRY COMPOTE

Makes 2 Cups
1 Tablespoon =
1/5 Fruit Exchange
12 Calories

C = 3  P = 0  F = 0

1 (10 ounce) package frozen blueberries, unsweetened
1 tablespoon lemon juice
½ cup apple juice concentrate
1-½ teaspoons cornstarch
1-½ teaspoons unflavored gelatin (½ envelope)

Partially thaw berries saving all the juice. In a small sauce pan combine the apple juice concentrate, cornstarch and gelatin. Cook over medium heat, stirring to dissolve until mixture comes to a full boil. Add the blueberries and simmer sauce about 10 minutes until berries are cooked. Cool and enjoy!

* Makes terrific filling for dessert crepes with a dollop of whipped cream.

* Pour blueberry mixture into blender if a smoother jam type is preferred. Do this while still warm and then reheat to a full boil to thicken again.

* Really good slightly warm to top ice cream or cornbread.

* This is delicious in homemade ice cream.

# BLACKBERRY JAM

Makes 2 Cups
1 Teaspoon Free
1 Tablespoon Equals
1/6 Fruit Exchange
10 Calories

C = 2.5  P = 0  F = 0

2 cups crushed blackberries, fully ripe
1/4 cup apple juice concentrate
1 tablespoon cornstarch

Measure crushed blackberries and juice into large sauce pan. Add concentrate and cornstarch. Stir well. Cook over medium heat, stirring constantly, until mixture comes to a full boil and thickens. Remove from heat and allow to cool to room temperature. Store in refrigerator.

* Delicious warm on waffles or french toast.

* Chilled this makes a great filling for a cake or jelly roll.

* Freeze berries in 2 cup bags so you can make fresh jam any time.

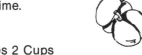

# PEACH JAM

Makes 2 Cups
1 Teaspoon Free
1 Tablespoon Equals
1/6 Fruit Exchange
10 Calories

C = 2.5  P = 0  F = 0

4 cups very ripe peaches, peeled and pitted
1 tablespoon lemon juice
1/4 cup apple juice concentrate
1 package powdered pectin
1/2 teaspoon fruit fresh

In a large sauce pan crush peaches. Add pectin, fruit fresh, concentrate and lemon juice. Stir over medium heat until mixture comes to a full boil. Boil one minute. Remove from heat and continue stirring for two additional minutes. Refrigerate.

* This freezes well.

* The riper the peaches — the more flavor they have.

# FRUIT BUTTER

10 dried apricots
½ cup raisins
2 medium apples, peeled and sliced
½ teaspoon cinnamon

1 Tablespoon Equals
⅓ Fruit Exchange
20 Calories

C = 5   P = 0   F = 0

Place apples in blender and blend about 30 seconds to form some liquid, add raisins and apricots and blend until thick and smooth.  Store in refrigerator.

Good on warm biscuits, toast or bagels with cream cheese.

## EASY STRAWBERRY JAM

Makes Approx. 2-½ Cups
1 Tablespoon Free
Fruit Exchange negligible
10 Calories

1 envelope unflavored gelatin
4 teaspoons tapioca
⅔ cup unsweetened white grape juice (undiluted)
2 teaspoons fresh lemon juice
2 cups mashed-fully ripe strawberries.

C = 2.5   P = 0   F = 0

Wash and mash berries.  Combine the gelatin, tapioca, grape juice and lemon juice in sauce pan. Stir and let stand 2 minutes. Over medium heat, stirring constantly, dissolve gelatin. (Takes about 2 minutes). Add the berries and bring to a boil, stirring constantly. Reduce heat and simmer uncovered about 5 minutes.  Cool and refrigerate.

# GRAPE JELLY

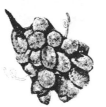

Makes 1-½ Cups
1 Teaspoon Free Exchange
10 Calories
$C = 2.5 \quad P = 0 \quad F = 0$

¼ cup water
1-½ cups (12 ounce can) grape juice concentrate, unsweetened
½ teaspoon lemon juice
1 envelope (1 tablespoon) gelatin

In a medium size sauce pan combine water, concentrate, lemon juice and gelatin. Let rest 5 minutes to soften gelatin. Put pan on stove over medium heat and bring to a full boil, stirring constantly. Pour into container and store in refrigerator.

* Remove from refrigerator at least 10 minutes before serving and allow to soften a bit. Best served at room temperature.

* Sticky sweet!

## PEAR-GRAPE JELLY

Substitute pear-grape concentrate for grape juice concentrate above. Sweet subtle flavor blend. Values remain the same as grape jelly.

## PLUM CONSERVE

Makes 1-½ Cups
1 Tablespoon Equals
⅓ Fruit Exchange
Fat Exchange negligible
25 Calories

$C = 5$  $P = 0$  $F = .05$

1 cup soft pitted prunes
½ cup apple juice concentrate
½ teaspoon cinnamon
¼ cup chopped walnuts

Place concentrate in blender on low speed to slush if not defrosted. Add prunes and blend until thick and creamy. Pour into "jam jar" and stir in chopped nuts.

* Super on hot toast or rolls.

## PRUNE SPREAD

Makes 1-¼ Cups
1 Tablespoon Equals
⅓ Fruit Exchange
20 Calories

$C = 5$  $P = 0$  $F = 0$

1 cup soft pitted prunes
½ cup apple juice concentrate
½ teaspoon cinnamon

Place concentrate in blender on low speed to slush if not defrosted. Add prunes and blend until thick and creamy. Refrigerate until needed.

* Great with peanut butter!

## QUICK PEACH BUTTER

Makes 2-½ Cups
2 Tablespoons Equals
¼ Fruit Exchange
Lean Meat negligible
15 Calories

C = 4  P = 0  F = 0

1 16 ounce can juice packed peaches, sliced
1 envelope unflavored gelatin
½ cup unsweetened apple juice
¼ teaspoon cinnamon or apple pie sauce

Drain peach juice into blender container. Add gelatin and let set 2 minutes to soften. Bring apple juice to boil while gelatin softens and add to container. Blend on high until dissolved. Add fruit & spice and blend until smooth. Taste and adjust spice. Refrigerate until set.

* Take out of refrigerator when beginning meal preparation and allow to come to room temperature to enhance flavor.
* Good spread for biscuits and toast.
* Yummy with peanut butter.

**QUICK APRICOT BUTTER:** Substitute juice packed apricots for peaches.
Values are the same as with peaches.

## DATE BUTTER

Makes 1 Cup
1 Tablespoon Equals
½ Fruit Exchange
30 Calories

1 cup chopped dates (not sugared)
½ cup water

$C = 7.5$   $P = 0$   $F = 0$

Place dates and water in covered saucepan.  Cook covered over very low heat until dates become very soft.  Pour into blender and blend until thick and smooth.  Store in refrigerator.

## DATE-NUT BUTTER

Makes 1 Cup
1 Tablespoon Equals
½ Fruit Exchange
Fat Exchange negligible
35 Calories

$C = 7.5$   $P = 0$   $F = .05$

Make date butter stirring in ¼ cup chopped walnuts after blending.

* If packaged chopped dates are unavailable without sugar – simply buy whole dates and chop.  Remove pits before cooking if they are still in the whole date.
* Date Butter and Date-Nut Butter are excellent fillings for cookies and breakfast rolls.
* Excellent sandwich filling for dark or nut breads mixed with cream cheese.
* Whipped butter doubles in volume.

# EASY APPLE JELLY

Makes 2-¼ Cups
1 Teaspoon Free
1 Tablespoon Equals
1/6 Fruit Exchange
10 Calories

C = 2.5  P = 0  F = 0

¼ cup apple juice concentrate
2 cups unsweetened apple juice
1 envelope (1 tablespoon) unflavored gelatin
1 teaspoon lemon juice

In a medium sized sauce pan combine all ingredients and bring to a full rolling boil, stirring constantly to dissolve gelatin and avoid scorching. Pour into container and cool to room temperature. Store in refrigerator.

# SPICY APPLE JELLY

For a spicy apple jelly follow easy apple jelly recipe above except add a spice bag tied in cheese cloth to the pan during cooking. For the spice bag use ¼ teaspoon cloves, dash of all-spice and ½ teaspoon cinnamon. Remove spice bag as soon as cooking is complete.

# CINNAMON-APPLE JELLY

Simply add a cinnamon stick to easy apple jelly during cooking.

## BOYSENBERRY SYRUP

Makes 1 Cup
1 Tablespoon
Free Exchange
8 Calories

C = 2   P = 0   F = 0

1 cup unsweetened boysenberry juice
1 teaspoon cornstarch
drop of vanilla

Combine berry juice and cornstarch in a small sauce pan. Cook over medium heat, stirring constantly, until "syrupy" thick and beginning to boil. Remove from heat and stir in drop of vanilla. Enjoy warm or cold. Refrigerate sauce to store.

* Delicious on waffles, pancakes, ice cream or custard.

## RASPBERRY SYRUP

Make boysenberry syrup above substituting bottled unsweetened raspberry juice for the boysenberry juice. Values remain the same.

* Drizzle a teaspoon of raspberry syrup over a canned peach half for a jiffy peach melba.

## APPLE SYRUP

Makes about 1-¾ cups
(approximately 2 tablespoons)
12 Servings
1 Serving Equals
½ Fruit Exchange
Bread negligible
30 Calories

$C = 7.5$  $P = 0$  $F = 0$

1 6 ounce can frozen apple juice concentrate, unsweetened
1-½ tablespoons cornstarch
1 cup cold water
¼ teaspoon cinnamon, nutmeg or apple pie spice

Mix cornstarch in ½ cup water until smooth. Combine cornstarch/water mix, remaining water and concentrate in saucepan. Cook over medium heat, stirring constantly, until syrup thickens. Season with spice to taste. Serve warm. Refrigerate leftovers – reheat before serving. Will keep up to 10 days.

* Good on pancakes, waffles, french toast or ice cream.

## SAUCY PINEAPPLE SYRUP

Serves 6
1 Serving Equals
½ Fruit Exchange
Bread Exchange negligible
30 Calories

$C = 7.5 \quad P = 0 \quad F = 0$

1 8 ounce can crushed pineapple in unsweetened juice
¾ to 1 tablespoon tapioca or cornstarch
¼ cup cold water
dash of cinnamon, if desired

Mix thickener in water. Combine all ingredients except cinnamon, in saucepan. Cook over medium-low heat until mixture thickens. Season with cinnamon if desired.

* Super on waffles – for a festive touch – sprinkle with unsweetened coconut.
* Tapioca makes the sauce a bit thicker and adds texture.
* For a smooth syrup, puree all ingredients in blender until smooth, transfer to saucepan and cook until thickened.

# MERINGUE

Serves 8
Exchanges negligible
10 Calories

$C = 1$  $P = 1$  $F = $ trace

3 egg whites
¼ teaspoon cream of tartar
4 teaspoons apple juice concentrate, thawed

Beat egg whites until frothy. Add cream of tartar and beat until stiff peaks form, but not dry. Add concentrate and continue beating until well blended. Top desired dish and bake in preheated 425 degree oven about 5 minutes until curls are lightly browned and set.

*   Make curls and swirls with back of spoon.

# ORANGE TOPPING

Makes 1 Cup
2 Tablespoons Equals
⅛ Lowfat Milk Exchange
15 Calories
Fruit Exchange negligible

$C = 2$  $P = 1$  $F = $ trace

⅓ cup non fat dry milk powder
⅓ cup ice cold orange juice

Mix milk powder and orange juice in small mixing bowl. Beat on high until stiff. Store covered in refrigerator.

*   Kids will enjoy fruit cups (fresh fruit served in half orange shells) frosted with orange topping and decorated with raisin faces! Adults will enjoy frosted fruit cups garnished with a sprig of mint.
*   Great on fruit salad.

61

## CHOCOLATE SYRUP

Makes 1-½ Cups
1 Tablespoon Equals
½ Fruit Exchange
30 Calories

C = 7.5  P = 0  F = 0

1 cup apple juice concentrate
½ cup grape juice concentrate
½ cup cocoa powder (unsweetened)
4 teaspoons vanilla

In a small sauce pan over medium heat combine juice concentrates, vanilla and cocoa. Stir with a wire whip until cocoa powder is dissolved and mix comes to a full rolling boil. Remove from heat as soon as syrup reaches the full boil stage.  Enjoy warm or cold. Refrigerate leftovers.

*   1-½ cups apple-grape or pear-grape concentrate may be substituted for the concentrates above.

## CHOCOLATE SAUCE

Makes 1-½ Cups
1 Tablespoon Equals
½ Fruit Exchange
35 Calories

C = 9  P = 0  F = 0

Make chocolate syrup above adding one tablespoon cornstarch.  Cook as directed stirring constantly to avoid sticking and scorching.  Cool to room temperature, cover and refrigerate.

62

# WHIPPED MAPLE BUTTER

Makes 1 Cup
1 Tablespoon Equals
1-½ Fat Exchanges
Fruit Exchange Negligible
65 Calories

$C = .5$  $P = 0$  $F = 7.5$

⅓ cup butter or margarine, room temperature
2 tablespoons apple juice concentrate
1 tablespoon maple flavoring

Cream butter or margarine in a deep bowl gradually adding apple juice concentrate while beating on high speed of electric mixer. Add flavoring 1 teaspoon at a time — tasting for maple strength as you go along. (Brands of extract vary in strength.) Beat until light and fluffy. Enjoy!

# PINEAPPLE-ORANGE BUTTER

½ cup butter or margarine, room temperature
1 tablespoon pineapple-orange concentrate, unsweetened
1 teaspoon grated orange rind

Mix as in Whipped Maple Butter above. Values are the same as Whipped Maple Butter above.

* Whipped Maple and Orange Butters are great on waffles, pancakes and french toast!

# APPLE-CRANBERRY SAUCE

1 cup cranberries
¼ cup apple juice concentrate
1-½ cup apple juice
1 tablespoon orange juice concentrate
2 tablespoons cornstarch

Serves 5
1 Serving Equals
1 Fruit Exchange
Starch/Bread Exchange negligible
60 Calories

C = 15  P = 0  F = 0

Wash berries and pick out any that are brown. Mix apple juice concentrate, apple juice, orange juice concentrate and cornstarch in saucepan stirring to mix and dissolve cornstarch. Stir in cranberries. Cook over medium heat until cranberries pop. Serve warm or cold.

* These are good with a cinnamon stick cooked in the sauce for a spicy flavor.
* Cranberries freeze well. In the Fall buy several bags and freeze in bags until time to cook.

## RASPBERRY SAUCE

Makes 1 Cup
2 Tablespoons Equals
¼ Fruit Exchange
15 Calories

C = 4  P = 0  F = 0

1 package (10 ounce) frozen, unsweetened raspberries, thawed
1 teaspoon cornstarch
2 tablespoons apple juice concentrate, thawed

In a small pan combine raspberries (and their juice), cornstarch and apple juice concentrate. Bring to a full boil over medium heat. Cook stirring constantly 2 minutes. Cool and refrigerate. Sauce continues to thicken as it cools.

# PIES

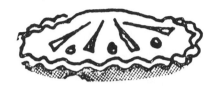

## PASTRY (PIE) CRUST

Serves 8
1 Serving (crust only) =
170 Calories
1 Bread Exchange
2 Fat Exchanges

C = 15  P = 3  F = 10

1 cup flour
dash of salt
⅓ cup shortening
2 tablespoons cold water

In a small bowl, mix flour and salt. Add shortening and cut into flour until particles are about the size of peas. Add water and mix with a fork until the dough forms a ball. Roll out on a lightly floured board or pastry canvas. If rolled very thin, makes enough for one 9 or 10 inch pie shell or an 8 inch 2 crust pie.

# GRAHAM CRACKER CRUST

Serves 6
1 Serving Equals
⅔ Bread Exchange
1 Fat Exchange
99 Calories

12 graham crackers (squares)
2 tablespoons melted butter or margarine

C = 10   P = 2   F = 5

Crush graham crackers.  Melt butter and mix with cracker crumbs.  Press into 8 inch pie plate.  Refrigerate 1 hour before filling with cool filling.  Bake 7-8 minutes at 350 degrees (until lightly brown and firm) allow to cool, if filling with warm filling.

* An easy way to crumb the crackers is in your blender or place crackers in large plastic baggie and roll with rolling pin until finely crushed.

# GRAHAM CRACKER-WALNUT CRUST

Serves 6
1 Serving Equals
¾ Bread Exchange
1-⅔ Fat Exchanges
130 Calories

1 cup graham cracker crumbs (12 squares)
7 teaspoons butter or margarine
⅓ cup finely chopped nuts

C = 10   P = 2   F = 8.33

Combine crumbs and nuts in 8 inch pie plate or spring form pan.  Melt butter or margarine and mix with crumbs.  Press into bottom or sides of pan.  Refrigerate 1 hour allowing butter to chill and set crust.  Fill as desired.

* Rich nutty flavor makes any dessert extra special.

# BLUEBERRY CREAM CHEESE PIE

Serves 8
1 Serving Equals
3 Fat Exchanges
⅔ Fruit Exchange
½ Bread Exchange
Milk negligible
215 Calories

$C = 17.5 \quad P = 1.5 \quad F = 10$

1 9 inch baked pastry shell (1 crust type) (page 65 )

1 1 pound can blueberries, juice or water pack
1 8-¾ ounce can crushed pineapple in pineapple juice
1 8 ounce package neufchatel cheese, room temperature
1 tablespoon milk
½ teaspoon vanilla
2 tablespoons cornstarch                    * Includes crust
dash of salt
½ teaspoon lemon juice
1 cup whipped cream

Drain fruits in separate bowls reserving juice. Blend neufchatel cheese, milk and vanilla. Stir in pineapple (reserve 2 tablespoons for garnish). Spread cheese-pineapple mixture in bottom of crust. Refrigerate. Measure pineapple juice and add enough blueberry liquid to equal 1-½ cups. Over medium heat stir juices, cornstarch and salt until thickened. Stir in blueberries and lemon juice. Cool. Pour over cheese layer. Chill. Top with whipped cream and garnish with reserved pineapple bits.

# PUMPKIN PIE

Serves 8
1 Serving Equals
1 Bread Exchange
2 Fat Exchanges
⅓ Medium Fat Meat Exchange
½ Vegetable Exchange
¾ Fruit Exchange
⅓ Whole Milk Exchange
290 Calories

$C = 33$  $P = 10$  $F = 13$

1 unbaked pie crust (page 65   )

3 eggs
1 (16 ounce) can pumpkin
¾ cup apple juice concentrate
¼ teaspoon salt
1-¼ teaspoon cinnamon
½ teaspoon ginger
¼ teaspoon cloves
1 can (12 ounce) evaporated milk

* Includes crust

Make one crust pie shell and line a 9 inch pie plate with deep sides.  Preheat oven to 425 degrees.  In a large bowl slightly beat eggs with a wire whip and add concentrate, salt and spices. Blend well.  Pour in evaporated milk and stir to blend.  Pour into unbaked pie shell and bake 15 minutes.  Without opening oven door — reduce oven temperature to 375 degrees and continue baking an additional 40-45 minutes or until a table knife inserted in the center comes out clean.

* Pumpkin pie is an anytime favorite with a dollop of whipped cream.

* This recipe may be doubled to make 2 pies successfully.

* Skim evaporated milk tends to make the pie a bit soft.

# PUMPKIN CHIFFON PIE

Serves 6
One Serving Equals
½ Bread Exchange
1 Fat Exchange
⅓ Medium Fat Meat Exchange
1 Fruit Exchange
½ Vegetable Exchange
175 Calories

C = 25  P = 5.5  F = 6

1 Graham Cracker Crust (page 66 )

2 eggs, separated
¾ cup apple juice concentrate, thawed
1-½ cups pumpkin
1 teaspoon cinnamon
½ teaspoon ginger
¼ teaspoon ground cloves
1 envelope unflavored gelatin
¼ cup cold water

* Includes crust

In a medium sized sauce pan beat together the egg yolks and apple juice concentrate with a wire whip. Stir in pumpkin and spices. Place pan over medium heat and cook stirring constantly until thick. Remove from heat. Dissolve gelatin in water and stir into warm pumpkin mixture. Refrigerate until partially set. Beat egg whites until stiff and fold into pumpkin until blended in. Pour into crust and refrigerate until serving time.

*   Festive with a dollop of whipped cream.

69

# CRUSTLESS PUMPKIN SQUARES

Serves 9
One Serving Equals
⅓ Medium Fat Meat Exchange
½ Vegetable Exchange
¾ Fruit Exchange
⅓ Whole Milk Exchange
125 Calories

C = 18   P = 6   F = 4

Make Pumpkin Pie Filling above and bake in lightly buttered 8" square baking dish. Test for doneness 35 minutes after turning the heat to 350 degrees.  Cool on wire rack and cut into 9 squares.  Refrigerate to store.

*   Serve topped with 1 tablespoon whipped cream.  F = 2.5   23 Calories.

# PUMPKIN MOUSSE

Serves 6
One Serving Equals
⅓ Medium Fat Meat Exchange
1 Fruit Exchange
½ Vegetable Exchange
95 Calories

C = 17.5   P = 4   F = 1

Spoon pumpkin chiffon pie filling into six individual serving bowls or fancy wine glasses and refrigerate until serving time.

# SUGARFREE APPLE PIE

Makes 8 Servings
1 Serving (including the crust) =
230 Calories
1 Fruit Exchange
1 Bread Exchange
2 Fat Exchanges

Pastry Crust for 8" 2 crust pie (page 65 )

$C = 30 \quad P = 3 \quad F = 10$

4 cups sliced peeled apples (sweet varieties are best)
½ cup frozen apple juice concentrate, undiluted
1-½ to 2 teaspoons tapioca, cornstarch or flour (see note)
½ teaspoon lemon juice, optional
½ to 1 teaspoon cinnamon, nutmeg or apple pie spice

Divide pastry into 2 parts and roll thin to fit an 8 or 9 inch plate. Set aside.

Mix apples, apple juice concentrate, thickener and spice and stir until apples are well-coated. Add lemon juice, if desired, to keep apples lighter-colored. Taste 1 piece of apple to check the spice. Pour into the pastry-lined pie pan and top with the second crust or pastry strips. Seal the edges and cut slits in the top crust to allow steam to escape. Bake at 425 degrees for 40-45 minutes, until golden brown. Serve warm or cold.

Note: Apples have some natural pectin, but a small amount of thickener seems necessary to "hold" the sweet concentrate of the apples for an even flavor.

# DEEP DISH APPLE PIE

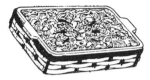

Serves 16
1 Serving Equals
1 Fruit Exchange
½ Bread Exchange
1 Fat Exchange
145 Calories

$C = 22.5$  $P = 1.5$  $F = 5$

Make sugar free apple pie — doubling the amount of the filling. Place in 9 x 13 baking dish. Roll out the pastry crust for 2 crust 8" pie into rectangle to top baking dish with crust sealing edges. Cut slits in top and bake at 425 degrees about 45 minutes until golden brown and bubbly.

Only has one crust – same great taste – fewer calories. Great for large groups. Generous servings.

* This pie is a real favorite and enjoyed by everyone!
* Great with a slice of cheddar cheese.
* Includes crust
* For a fancy top crust roll the pastry dough into a 9 x 13 inch rectangle and cut into one inch wide strips the long way of the dough. Secure strips to one end of baking pan over apples and twist before securing on opposite end.

# PEACH PIE

Serves 8
1 Serving Equals
½ Fruit Exchange
1 Bread Exchange
2 Fat Exchanges
200 Calories

C = 22.5  P = 3  F = 10

Pastry Crust for 8" 2 crust pie (page 65 )

1 16 ounce can sliced peaches canned in fruit juice undrained
2 tablespoons quick cooking tapioca
2 drops almond extract
½ teaspoon cinnamon

\* Includes crust

Divide pastry into 2 parts and roll them to fit an 8 inch pie plate. Line bottom of pie plate and set aside.

Preheat oven to 425 degrees. Mix peaches and juice, tapioca, almond extract and cinnamon. Pour into prepared unbaked pie crust and top with second crust. Seal the edges and cut slits in top to allow steam to escape. Bake for 40-45 minutes in pre-heated oven – until golden brown. Serve warm or cold.

# BLUEBERRY PEACH PIE

Serves 8
1 Serving Equals
¾ Fruit Exchange
1 Bread Exchange
2 Fat Exchanges
220 Calories

C = 28  P = 3  F = 10

Pastry crust for 2 crust 9" pie (page 65 )

1 cup unsweetened blueberries – fresh or drained canned or frozen
16 ounce can sliced peaches canned in fruit juice, undrained
2-½ – 3 tablespoons tapioca
¾ teaspoon cinnamon

* Includes crust

Preheat oven to 425 degrees.  Line bottom of pie plate with crust.  Mix all filling ingredients.  Pour into prepared botton crust.  Top with remaining crust.  Seal edges. Cut slits (I like to make a tree shape) in top crust to allow steam to escape. Bake 40-50 minutes until golden brown.  Remove from oven and cool on rack.

*  Delicious warm.

# EARLY AMERICAN PEAR PIE

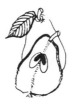

Serves 8
1 Serving Equals
½ Fruit Exchange
1 Bread Exchange
2 Fat Exchanges
200 Calories

C = 22.5  P = 3  F = 10

Pastry Crust for 8" 2 crust pie (page 65 )

1 16 ounce can pears canned in fruit juice, undrained
2 tablespoons quick cooking tapioca
¾ teaspoon cinnamon or nutmeg

* Includes crust

Divide pastry into 2 parts and roll thin to fit an 8 inch pie plate. Line bottom of pie plate and set aside.

Preheat oven to 425 degrees. Slice pear halves. Mix pears and juice, tapioca and spice. Pour into prepared unbaked pie shell and top with second crust. Seal the edges and cut slits in the top to allow the steam to escape. Bake for 40-45 minutes in pre-heated oven until golden brown. Serve warm or cold.

# RAISIN PIE

Serves 8
1 Serving Equals
1 Bread Exchange
2 Fat Exchanges
1-½ Fruit Exchanges
265 Calories

C = 39  P = 3  F = 10

*with nuts add 1 fat exchange,
45 calories and 5 grams fat

Pastry Crust for 8 inch pie (page 65 )

1-½ cups seedless raisins
½ cup boiling apple juice
1 cup boiling water
1-½ tablespoons flour or cornstarch
1-½ teaspoons grated lemon rind
2 tablespoons lemon juice
½ cup nuts (optional)*

* Includes crust

Make pastry for 2 crust pie. Line bottom of 8" pie plate with half crust. Set aside. Preheat oven to 425 degrees. In small saucepan cook raisins in water and apple juice (about 5 minutes) until tender. Stir in flour or cornstarch and stir constantly (about 2 minutes) until thickened. Remove from heat and add remaining ingredients. Pour hot filling into unbaked pastry shell. Top with remaining crust. Seal edges and cut vents to allow steam to escape. Bake 30-40 minutes – until golden brown.

* A Thanksgiving classic.
* If you like a spicy fruit filling – add cinnamon, nutmeg, or apple pie spice to taste.

# SOUR CREAM RAISIN PIE

Serves 8
1 Serving Equals
With Pastry Crust
1-1/2 Bread Exchange
1 Fruit Exchange
1/4 Milk Exchange
4 Fat Exchanges
380 Calories
C = 40.5  P = 6.5  F = 21

1 8" baked pastry crust (page 65 )
or graham cracker crust (page 66 )

Serves 8
1 Serving Equals
With Graham Cracker Crust
1 Bread Exchange
1 Fruit Exchange
1/4 Milk Exchange
2-3/4 Fat Exchanges
265 Calories
C = 33  P = 5  F = 13.75

1 cup raisins
1 egg
2 cups skim milk
1/2 cup cornstarch
2 cups sour cream
3/4 teaspoon cinnamon
2 teaspoons vanilla

In a small saucepan over medium-low heat combine egg, milk and cornstarch. Cook, stirring consistently for 5 minutes. Add raisins, continue to stir constantly, and cook an additional 3-5 minutes until thick and creamy. Remove from heat. (The raisins will be tender plump and the custard slightly sweet.) Stir in cinnamon and vanilla and cool to room temperature. Stir in sour cream and mix well. Pour into pie crust and refrigerate until firm.

* Do not cool raisin/custard mixture in the refrigerator before adding sour cream or custard mixture will be slightly lumpy and a bit watery.

* In the pastry crust it is a "pie dessert" — in the lower calorie graham cracker crust it is more of a "cheesecake" type goodie.

# PARADISE PIE

Serves 8
1 Serving Equals
½ Bread Exchange
2 Fat Exchanges
1-½ Fruit Exchanges
185 Calories

C = 22.5  P = 1  F = 10

Crust
½ recipe pastry crust (page 65 )

Filling
1 orange, peeled and chopped
1 20 oz. can crushed pineapple in pineapple juice
2 tablespoons tapioca or cornstarch
5 tablespoons light or golden raisins

\* Includes crust

Topping
1 cup whipped cream

Prepare pastry crust for 1 crust pie – pricking bottom and sides with fork. Bake in 425 degree oven 7-8 minutes until lightly browned. Remove from oven and allow to cool. Combine filling ingredients in medium sauce pan. Simmer over low heat, stirring occasionally, until mixture thickens (20-25 minutes). Cool to room temperature and pour into cooled pastry shell. Chill and top with whipped cream.

\* Cream may be flavored with a drop of orange extract or pineapple flavoring, if desired.

78

# FRESH RASPBERRY PIE

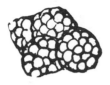

Serves 6
(Generous Servings)
1 Serving Equals
⅔ Fruit Exchange
⅔ Bread Exchange
1 Fat Exchange
145 Calories

C = 20   P = 2   F = 5

1 Graham Cracker Crust  (page 66)

¾ cup apple juice or apple berry juice
1 tablespoon cornstarch                    * Includes crust
3 cups fresh raspberries

Rinse raspberries and put ½ cup berries in small sauce pan, reserving other 2-½ cups. Mash berries and add apple juice and cornstarch.  Cook over medium heat, stirring constantly until mixture comes to a full rolling boil.  Remove from heat and allow to cool.  Gently fold raspberries into glaze and spoon mixture into graham cracker crust.  Refrigerate until serving time.

*   Delicious with a dollop of whipped cream.

*   The glazed raspberries are also wonderful on puddings or waffles.

# STRAWBERRY CHIFFON PIE

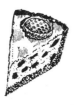

Serves 8
1 Serving Equals
2 Fat Exchanges
½ Bread Exchange
⅔ Fruit Exchange
Meat negligible
170 Calories

$C = 17.5$   $P = 1.5$   $F = 10$

1 8 inch baked pastry shell (1 crust type) (page 65 )

2-½ cups fully ripe fresh strawberries
1 envelope unflavored gelatin
¾ cup apple or apple-pear juice
1 teaspoon lemon juice
2 egg whites
1 cup whipped cream

* Includes crust

Crush strawberries and add ¼ cup apple or apple-pear juice. Soften gelatin in remaining ½ cup juice and dissolve over low heat.  Allow juice/gelatin to cool slightly and mix with berries and lemon juice. Chill, stirring occasionally until partially set. (It's important that the gelatin be just the right consistency – partially set but still pourable).  Beat egg. whites to form soft peaks. Fold beaten egg whites into strawberry mixture, then whipped cream.  Chill until strawberry filling mounds but is not firm.  Pile high into cooled pie shell and chill until firm.

Pretty trimmed with whipped cream stars and fresh berry halves.  For special occasions trim with berry halves and silver leaves.

# FROZEN STRAWBERRY PIE

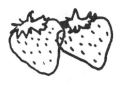

Serves 8
1 Serving Equals
2-¾ Fat Exchanges
½ Bread Exchange
⅓ Fruit Exchange
185 Calories

C = 12.5  P = 1.5  F = 13.75

* Includes crust

1 graham cracker crust (page 66 )

1 8 ounce package neufchatel cheese, room temperature
1 cup sour cream (not imitation)
2 10 ounce packages non sugared frozen strawberries, defrosted

Blend cheese and sour cream.  Reserve ½ cup berries and set aside.  Mix remaining berries and any juice in cheese/sour cream base.  Pour into crust and freeze until firm.  Remove from freezer 5 minutes before serving.  Cut into wedges and spoon 1 tablespoon reserved berries and juice over each wedge.

*  Great hot weather dessert – cool and slightly tangy.


## FROZEN BLUEBERRY PIE

Substitute frozen blueberries for strawberries.

# FRESH GLAZED PEACH PIE

Serves 6
(Generous Servings)
1 Serving Equals
1 Fruit Exchange
⅔ Bread Exchange
1 Fat Exchange
150 Calories

C = 25  P = 2  F = 5

1 Graham Cracker Crust  (page 66)

1 cup apple juice, peach juice or pear juice
1 tablespoon cornstarch
2 drops almond extract
2 cups sliced fresh ripe peaches, peeled

\* Includes crust

Mix juice and cornstarch in small sauce pan.  Cook over medium heat, stirring constantly until glaze becomes thick and begins to boil.  Remove from heat and stir in almond.  Cool to room temperature.  Stir glaze into peaches and gently mix with rubber scraper to coat.  Pour into pie shell.  Refrigerate two hours before serving.

\*  Delicious served with a dollop of whipped cream.

# FRENCH BERRY GLAZE PIE

Serves 8
1 Serving Equals
½ Bread Exchange
2 Fat Exchanges
¾ Fruit Exchange
170 Calories

C = 17.5  P = 1.5  F = 10

1 baked 9" pie shell, cooled (½ pie crust recipe) (**page 65** )

1 quart fresh sliced strawberries, raspberries, blackberries or blueberries
1 cup apple juice
2-½ – 3 tablespoons cornstarch
1 8 ounce package  **neufchatel cheese**, room temperature

* Includes crust

Wash and drain berries, slicing strawberries only. Simmer 1 cup berries in ⅔ cup apple juice 3 minutes (sweeter if these berries are crushed). Blend in cornstarch and stir constantly 1 minute over medium high heat – until mixture thickens. Remove from heat and cool. Spread softened cheese in baked shell. Top with 2-½ cups berries (save ½ cup to garnish). Cover with cooked fruit mixture and garnish with berries. Refrigerate 2-3 hours until firm. Enjoy!

*  Luscious and rich with a dollop of whipped cream.

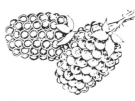

# JELLED BERRY PIE

Serves 8
1 Serving Equals
⅔ Fruit Exchange
½ Bread Exchange
1 Fat Exchange
Meat negligible
125 Calories

$C = 17.5$  $P = 1.5$  $F = 5$

½ recipe pastry crust – baked – prepared for 1 crust pie ( **page 65** )

2 cups frozen unsweetened strawberries, blueberries or raspberries
1 cup unsweetened grape juice (red for strawberries & raspberries – White or Purple for blueberries)
1 envelope unflavored gelatin                    Includes crust

Defrost berries but do not drain. Mash ½ cup berries to draw more juice and mix with remaining whole berries and berry liquid. Mix gelatin and grape juice in small sauce pan and let set 2 minutes. Bring to a boil stirring to dissolve gelatin. Mix juice/gelatin mix in berries. Let cool to room temperature and pour in shell. Refrigerate until set. Top with a dollop of whipped cream.

* This filling may also be used as a topping for custard, puddings or cheese cake.

# "NO BAKE" YOGURT FRUIT PIE

Serves 6
1 Serving Equals
1/2 Fruit Exchange
1 Fat Exchange
1/2 Bread Exchange
1/6 Milk Exchange
125 Calories

1 Graham Cracker Crust (page 66 )

$C = 17 \quad P = 3 \quad F = 5$

2-1/2 cups strawberries or 2 cups raspberries
1/3 cup white grape juice
2 envelopes unflavored gelatin (2 tablespoons)
1 cup plain non-fat yogurt
2 teaspoons vanilla

Includes crust

1/4 teaspoon cinnamon (if desired with raspberries)

In a small saucepan sprinkle gelatin on grape juice and heat to dissolve. Set aside. Place one half cup of berries in the bottom of the graham cracker crust and distribute evenly. (I like to save one berry out to garnish the center of the finished pie.) Place remaining berries, yogurt vanilla, and cinnamon in blender and puree. Add juice/gelatin and whip until blended. Pour filling over berries in shell. Garnish with whole berry and refrigerate at least 2 hours before serving. Store in the refrigerator.

# EASY APPLE DUMPLINGS

Serves 4
1 Serving Equals
1 Starch Bread Exchange
1 Fat Exchange
1-½ Fruit Exchanges
215 Calories

C = 37.5   P = 3   F = 5

4 flaky refrigerator biscuits
2 apples, peeled, cored and cut in half
¼ cup raisins
¼ teaspoon cinnamon or apple pie spice
1 cup apple juice
2 teaspoons butter, melted
½ teaspoon vanilla

Preheat oven to 375 degrees. Roll the refrigerator biscuits out into 4 six inch circles. Place one half apple cut side up on each biscuit round. Put 1 tablespoon raisins in center and 1 tablespoon apple juice. Fold the edges of the biscuit together over the apple and pinch securely together. Place in 8 inch square baking dish. Combine apple juice, vanilla, spice and melted butter. Pour apple juice sauce in baking dish. Bake about 40 minutes basting every 10 minutes until dumplings are light brown and apple is soft. Serve warm.

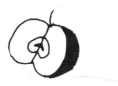

# CAKES AND COOKIES

## BASIC CAKE LAYER

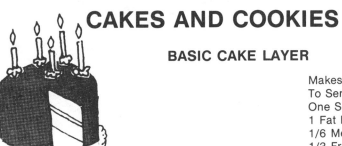

Makes 1 Layer
To Serve 12
One Serving Equals
1 Fat Exchange
1/6 Medium Fat Meat Exchange
1/3 Fruit Exchange
1/2 Bread Exchange
120 Calories
C = 13   P = 3   F = 6

To Serve 8
One Serving Equals
1-1/2 Fat Exchange
1/4 Medium Fat Meat Exchange
1/2 Fruit Exchange
3/4 Bread Exchange
180 Calories
C = 19   P = 4   F = 9.5

¼ cup butter or margarine, room temperature
2 eggs
1 teaspoon vanilla
½ cup apple or pineapple juice
   concentrate, thawed
1 cup flour
½ teaspoon baking soda
½ teaspoon baking powder

Measure dry ingredients (flour by dip-level method) and mix together and set aside. Beat together butter or margarine, eggs and vanilla until well blended. On medium mixer speed or by hand alternately add concentrate and dry ingredients until mixed. Beat one additional minute. Pour into prepared cake pan 20 to 25 minutes

* This makes a 1 inch to 1-½ inch thick layer. Has great cake texture and flavor but does not get as "high" as a "sugar prepared cake" due to the lack of extra bulk sugar provides.

* For special occasions I prefer to bake this in an 8 inch square pan and split it into 2 layers 4" x 8" making a bar cake. I often then split each layer and fill between to make a 4 layer torte type cake.

# PINEAPPLE UPSIDE DOWN CAKE

Serves 9
1 Serving Equals
1 Bread Exchange
Milk negligible
½ Fruit Exchange
1-⅔ Fat Exchanges
Medium Fat Meat negligible
185 Calories

C = 22.5   P = 4   F = 8.33

Topping:
1 20 ounce can crushed juice packed pineapple, drained — reserve juice. *See note.
½ teaspoon cinnamon or nutmeg
1 tablespoon melted butter or margarine
Cake:
1-½ cups flour
½ teaspoon cinnamon
½ teaspoon baking soda
1 teaspoon baking powder
½ cup reserved pineapple juice
2 tablespoons skim or low fat milk
1 egg
¼ cup vegetable oil

*   2 tablespoons whipped cream equals
    1 fat exchange,
    45 calories,

    C = 0  P = 0  F = 5.

Preheat oven to 350 degrees. Lightly grease 8" square or 8" round cake dish. Melt butter and mix with well drained pineapple and spice. Spread evenly in bottom of pan. Combine flour, cinnamon, baking powder, baking soda in mixing bowl. Add egg, oil, milk and pineapple juice and beat well. Pour batter over pineapple. Bake 28-30 minutes. Cool about 15 minutes (will still be warm) and carefully invert onto serving plate. Serve warm with whipped cream.
Note: Use reserved juice for the cake batter. There should be the ½ cup juice needed to sweeten the cake. If there is not quite enough juice you can use a bit more milk to make the ½ cup.

# SPICY BANANA NUT CAKE

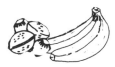

Serves 12
1 Serving Equals
¼ Medium Fat Meat Exchange
1 Bread Exchange
⅓ Fruit Exchange
2-½ Fat Exchanges
235 Calories

$C = 20$  $P = 5$  $F = 14$

½ cup butter or margarine, room temperature
3 small ripe bananas (about 1 cup)
3 eggs
¾ cup water
2 cups flour
2 teaspoons baking powder
1 teaspoon baking soda
¼ teaspoon salt
¾ teaspoon cinnamon
¾ cup chopped walnuts
Preheat oven to 350 degrees.  Lightly grease and flour 9 x 13 pan and set aside.

Mash bananas in large mixing bowl and mix with butter or margarine.  Add eggs and water mixing well.  Mix in flour, baking powder, baking soda, salt, and cinnamon until smooth.  Stir in chopped nuts.  Pour into prepared pan.  Bake 20-25 minutes until wooden pick inserted in center comes out clean.

* Excellent with French pastry icing or a dollop of whipped cream.

* Orange French pastry icing makes a delightful flavor combination.

# PINEAPPLE COFFEE-CAKE

Serves 12
1 Serving Equals
Meat negligible
1 Bread Exchange
½ Fruit Exchange
1-¾ Fat Exchange
190 Calories

C = 22.5  P = 3  F = 8.75

¼ cup butter or margarine
2 eggs
⅔ cup unsweetened pineapple juice
2 cups flour
½ teaspoon baking soda
2 teaspoons baking powder
½ teaspoon salt
1-½ cups juice packed crushed pineapple, drained
1 cup unsweetened shredded or flaked coconut
½ teaspoon cinnamon
¼ cup chopped walnuts

Preheat oven to 350 degrees. Lightly grease and flour a 9 inch square baking pan and set aside. Cream together eggs, butter and pineapple juice. Add flour, baking soda, baking powder and salt. Beat 2 minutes. Gently mix in 1 cup of drained, crushed pineapple and coconut. Pour into prepared pan. Sprinkle remaining pineapple over top. Mix nuts and cinnamon and top cake batter. Bake approximately 25 minutes until center springs back when lightly touched and cake is golden.

Yummy warm with a dollop of whipped cream!

# ORANGE DATE SNACKIN' CAKE

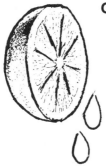

Makes 1 small loaf
12 Slices
1 Slice Equals
115 Calories
Milk negligible
Meat negligible
½ Fruit Exchange
1 Fat Exchange
½ Bread Exchange

C = 15   P = 1.5   F = 5

10 large pitted dates, chopped to make about ½ cup
½ cup non fat dry milk
¼ cup butter or stick-type margarine, softened
1 egg
¾ cup orange juice
1 cup flour
1-½ teaspoons baking powder
½ teaspoon salt

Cream butter or margarine with dry milk powder. Add egg and orange juice and beat well. Stir in flour, baking powder and salt. Mix until well blended. Stir in chopped dates, mixing well until evenly distributed.

Preheat oven to 325 degrees. Bake in a lightly greased loaf pan for 45-50 minutes, until cake appears done and a wooden toothpick inserted in center comes out clean. Cool and slice.

* This is a heavy type cake and is good in lunches as it can be eaten easily with fingers.

91

# CARROT CAKE

Serves 12
1 Serving Equals
⅓ Medium Fat Meat Exchange
1-¼ Bread Exchange
½ Fruit Exchange
½ Vegetable Exchange
2 Fat Exchanges
250 Calories

$C = 28$   $P = 7.33$   $F = 11$

½ cup butter or margarine, room temperature
3 eggs
1 cup unsweetened pineapple juice
2-½ cups flour
1 teaspoon baking soda
2 teaspoons baking powder
½ teaspoon salt
1 teaspoon nutmeg
1-½ teaspoons cinnamon
3 cups grated carrots
1 cup unsweetened crushed pineapple, drained

Preheat oven to 350 degrees. Lightly grease and flour 9 x 13 baking pan and set aside. Cream eggs and butter. Stir in pineapple juice. Add remaining ingredients except carrot and pineapple and beat 2 minutes. Stir in carrots and well drained pineapple. Pour into pan and spread out evenly. Bake 30-35 minutes until center springs back lightly when touched and cake is lightly browned. Cool on wire rack.

* Excellent frosted with cream cheese or French pastry icing.

# FRESH FRUIT CAKE

Serves 8
1 Serving Equals
¼ Medium Fat Meat Exchange
½ Bread Exchange
⅔ Fruit Exchange
100 Calories

C = 18   P = 4   F = 1.5

2 eggs, separated
¼ cup apple juice concentrate
¾ cup flour
2 teaspoons baking powder
2-¼ cups blueberries or sliced fresh peaches
     or blackberries or a combination
     of peaches and blueberries
¼ teaspoon cinnamon

Preheat oven to 375 degrees. Beat egg whites until stiff peaks form, add cinnamon and set aside. In another bowl beat together egg yolks, apple juice concentrate, flour and baking powder. Add fruit until coated with batter. Fold in egg whites until blended through. Pour into an 8 inch non-stick baking pan. Bake 15 to 20 minutes until firm and golden brown.

*   Use firm fresh fruit — canned fruit makes the crispy cake soggy.

*   Good dessert to serve warm and easy enough to bake while dinner cooks.

# WON TON CINNAMON COOKIES

Makes 40 Cookies
2 Cookies Equal
1/6 Bread/Starch Exchange
1/2 Fat Exchange
Fruit Negligible
35 Calories

C = 2.5   P = .5   F = 2.5

20 won ton skins
3 tablespoons butter or margarine, softened
1 tablespoon apple juice concentrate
½ teaspoon cinnamon

Preheat oven to 375 degrees.  Beat butter or margarine, apple juice concentrate and cinnamon together until light and fluffy.  Lightly butter each won ton and cut in half.  Place on an unbaked cookie sheet and bake 5 to 6 minutes, until crisp and golden brown. Remove from oven and cool on racks.

*   May use 5 egg roll wrappers and cut into quarters.

# BANANA WHIPPED CREAM ROLL

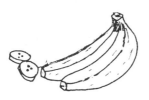

Serves 8
1 Serving Equals
½ Fruit Exchange
⅓ Medium Fat Meat Exchange
¼ Starch/Bread
1-½ Fat Exchange
150 Calories

C = 17   P = 4   F = 9.5

1 tablespoon pineapple juice concentrate
3 eggs separated
2 teaspoons vanilla
¼ cup flour
¼ teaspoon cream of tartar

For pan:
1 teaspoon butter or margarine

Filling:
1-½ cups whipped cream
2 (9 inch) bananas, sliced in ¼" rounds

Preheat oven to 325 degrees. Seperate eggs and put into mixing bowls. Beat concentrate, egg yolks and vanilla until thick and lemon colored. Gently fold flour into egg yolks one third at a time. Wash beaters. In the other bowl beat egg whites until foamy. Add cream of tartar and beat until very stiff. Gently fold egg whites into yolk mixture. Pour batter on to a buttered wax paper lined jelly roll pan (8" x 12" approximately) and bake about 15 minutes – should be lightly brown and firm to the touch. Immediately loosen edges of cake with a sharp knife and flip cake on to a clean (flour sack type) cotton dish towel. Peel off waxed paper and roll cake beginning at the small end. Let cool completely at room temperature while still in towel. Gently unroll. Spread evenly with whipped cream and cover cream with banana slices. Re-roll gently and refrigerate until serving. "Saw" into slices with a sharp knife. Enjoy!

# JELLY ROLL

Serves 8
1 Serving Equals
½ Fruit Exchange
⅓ Medium Fat Meat Exchange
¼ Starch Bread Exchange
80 Calories
$C = 11$  $P = 4$  $F = 2$

Make cake for banana whipped cream roll. Cool completely. Fill with 1 cup blackberry jam (page 51). Carefully re-roll. Refrigerate until shortly before serving time.

# ALMOND ANGEL KISSES

Makes 36 Cookies
1 Cookie Equals
⅔ Fat Exchange
Fruit is negligible
Meat is negligible
35 Calories

$C = 1$  $P = 0$  $F = 3.33$

3 egg whites
¼ teaspoon cream of tartar
2 tablespoons apple juice concentrate
1 drop almond extract
1-½ cup ground almonds (unsalted)

Beat egg whites until foamy. Gradually add cream of tartar beating until stiff. Beat in apple juice concentrate. Add drop of extract. Gently fold in nuts. Drop by teaspoons to form kisses on cookie sheet lined with baking parchment. Bake at 325 degrees until lightly browned 10-15 minutes. Cool completely before covering.

Walnuts and a dash of cinnamon may be substituted for almonds and extract.

# REFRIGERATOR COOKIES

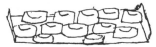

Makes 64 Cookies
2 Cookies Equal
1-¼ Fat Exchanges
1/6 Fruit Exchange
1/6 Bread Exchange
Meat Exchange negligible
80 Calories

$C = 5 \quad P = .05 \quad F = 6.25$

½ cup butter or margarine
1 egg
2 teaspoons vanilla
1 teaspoon baking powder
dash of salt
1 cup flour
1 cup chopped-unsugared dates
1 cup shredded coconut
1 cup chopped walnuts or pecans

Cream butter, egg and vanilla until mixed and fluffy. Beat in dry ingredients gradually mixing well after each addition. Mix in dates, coconut and ½ cup nuts. Form dough into two 1-½ inch logs. Roll logs in remaining nuts (¼ cup each). Wrap in waxed paper and chill (or freeze) until firm enough to slice. Preheat oven to 350 degrees. Slice cookies ¼"-⅜" thick and place on non stick cookie sheet. Bake 8-10 minutes until light golden brown. Cool on wire racks.

* A nice light, sweet, and crunchy cookie with a buttery richness.

# ORANGE RAISIN DROP COOKIES

33 Cookies
2 Cookies Equal
Meat Exchange negligible
⅔ Bread Exchange
⅔ Fat Exchange
⅓ Fruit Exchange
105 Calories
C = 15  P = 2.5  F = 3.33

1-¾ cups flour
2 teaspoons baking powder
¼ teaspoon salt
½ teaspoon cinnamon
¾ cup orange juice
½ teaspoon grated orange rind (if desired for a more distinct orange flavor)
7 tablespoons vegetable oil
1 egg
½ cup chopped walnuts or pecans
½ cup raisins

Preheat oven to 375 degrees. Combine all ingredients and mix well. Drop by heaping teaspoons onto ungreased – no stick – cookie sheet. Bake 12-15 minutes until firm and lightly brown. Cool on wire rack.

# APPLESAUCE BARS

Makes 16 Bars
1 Bar Equals
½ Fruit Exchange
1 Fat Exchange
¾ Bread Exchange
Medium Fat Meat negligible
135 Calories

C = 18.75   P = 3.5   F = 5.3

½ cup applesauce
½ cup apple juice
3 eggs
¼ cup butter or margarine
2 cups flour
½ teaspoon salt
1 teaspoon baking soda
2 teaspoons baking powder
½ teaspoon nutmeg
1-½ teaspoons cinnamon
¼ cup chopped walnuts
¾ cup raisins

Preheat oven to 350 degrees. Grease and flour an 8" square pan. In medium mixing bowl beat applesauce, apple juice, eggs and butter until well blended. Add flour, salt, baking soda, baking powder, nutmeg and cinnamon. Beat on medium speed 2 minutes, scraping sides often. Stir in nuts and raisins. Bake 25-30 minutes until a pick inserted in center comes out clean. Cool before cutting.

* Yummy with a dollop of whipped cream or topped with French pastry icing.

## MINI-COOKIE TARTS

Makes 24 Cookies
2 Cookies Equals
3-⅓ Fat Exchanges
Medium Fat Meat negligible
⅓ Fruit Exchange
⅔ Bread Exchange
230 Calories

½ cup butter or margarine, room temperature

$C = 15 \quad P = 2 \quad F = 17.5$

1 3 ounce package neufachtel cream cheese, room temperature
1-¼ cup flour
8 teaspoons apple juice concentrate
1 tablespoon butter or margarine, melted
1 cup chopped walnuts or pecans
¼ cup chopped dates
2 eggs, slightly beaten
½ teaspoon vanilla

Preheat oven to 350 degrees. Mix butter, cream cheese and flour to form soft dough. Make into 24 balls. Press 1 ball in each individual tart mold to form 1-½" inch shells. Set pastry shells aside. In small sauce pan melt butter over low heat. Remove pan from stove. Add apple juice concentrate, nuts, dates, and vanilla. Stir in beaten eggs, mix well. Spoon into unbaked prepared shells. Bake for 20-25 minutes until lightly browned and puffy. * Rich and flaky.

* Beautiful holiday cookies. * Make holiday cookies with a cookie press.

## DESSERT TARTS

* These can be baked in 12 individual tart pans. Per serving values are same as for 2 mini-cookie tart serving. Individual dessert tarts are wonderful served warm with a dollop of whipped cream.

## SOUR CREAM ROLL UPS

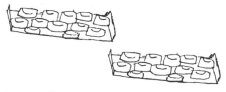

2 cups flour
1 cup butter or margarine, room temperature
¾ cup sour cream
1 egg yolk
1 cup chopped dates
1 cup water
¾ cup chopped walnuts
1 tablespoon grated orange peel

Makes 48 cookies
2 Cookies Equal
Meat negligible
½ Bread Exchange
2-½ Fat Exchanges
⅓ Fruit Exchange
175 Calories

C = 12.5  P = 1.5  F = 12.5

Cut soft butter or margarine into flour until mixture resembles corn meal. Add sour cream and egg yolk. Divide into 4 balls – wrap and refrigerate 2 hours. While dough chills combine dates and water in a sauce pan. Cook over medium heat until thick sauce forms. Remove from heat and stir in nuts and peel. Cool. To make cookies take one ball of chilled dough at a time and roll as for pie crust into a 10"-12" circle. Spread ¼ of filling on dough and cut into 12 pie shaped wedges. (I like to use a ravioli cutter for fancy edges). Roll each cookie from outside of circle to center and place point end down on ungreased cookie sheet. Bake in preheated 375 degree oven on top rack 20-25 minutes. Watch carefully as these brown easily. If browning too soon turn oven down a little or bake on double cookie sheet. Cool completely on wire racks. Cover and store in air tight tins.

* Flaky and tender.
* Our all year round favorite.     101

# RASPBERRY FILLED COOKIES

Makes 48 Cookies
2 Cookies Equal
Meat Negligible
½ Bread Exchange
2-½ Fat Exchange
Fruit Negligible
155 Calories

$C = 7.5$   $P = 1.5$   $F = 12.5$

2 cups flour
1 cup butter or margarine, room temperature
¾ cup sour cream
1 egg yolk
1 cup sugar free raspberry jam

Cut soft butter or margarine into flour until mixture resembles corn meal. Add sour cream and egg yolk. Mix well, divide into 4 balls — wrap and refrigerate 2 hours. (I often wrap 2 balls well and freeze at this point to bake later). To make cookies reheat oven to 375 degrees and take one ball of chilled dough at a time and roll as for pie crust into a 100" x 12" circle. Spread ¼ cup sugar free raspberry (or sugar free jam of choice) on dough and cut into 12 pie shaped wedges. (I like to use a ravioli cutter for fancy edges. Roll each cookie from the outside to the center. Place point down on cookie sheet. Bake on top oven rack about 20-25 minutes. Watch carefully — these brown easily. Cool completely on wine racks. Cover and store in airtight tins.

A rich sweet cookie.

## TART COOKIES

Roll dough into a 12 inch square. Spread one half square with ¼ cup sugar free raspberry jam and fold over dough to form a lid. Cut into 12 squares with a ravioli cutter to seal the edges. Prick each cookie in the center with tines of a fork so the steam can escape. Bake as above.

# FLAKEY "FIGGY" BARS

1 recipe pastry (pie) crust (page 65 )

Filling — 3/4 cup dried figs, chopped
2/3 cup water
1/2 teaspoon lemon juice
1 teaspoon vanilla

Makes 16 Bars
1 Bar Equals
1/2 Fruit Exchange
1/2 Bread Exchange
1 Fat Exchange
115 Calories

C = 15  P = 1.5  F = 5

Prepare pastry crust and divide in half. Roll one half into an 8 x 8 inch square and line the bottom of an 8 inch square baking pan. Roll the other half into an 8 x 8 inch square and set aside. In a small saucepan mix filling ingredients and simmer 20-25 minutes. Beat smooth with a wooden spoon. Place warm filling on pastry in pan and spread evenly. Cover with the remaining 8 x 8 pastry crust. With the tines of a fork prick through the pastry forming 16 squares. This allows the steam to escape and the cookies will be easy to cut and remove from the pan without crumbling to bits.

Bake in a preheated 425 degree oven 30-35 minutes until light golden brown. Cool in the pan on a wine rack. Cut into squares with a sharp knife.

# FLAKEY DATE BARS

Substitute 3/4 cup chopped unsugared dates for figs in Flaky "Figgy" Bars. Values the same as for recipe above.

# CHEESE COOKIES

Makes 96 Cookies
2 Cookies Equals
½ Fat Exchange
1/6 Bread Exchange
⅓ High Fat Meat Exchange
70 Calories

C = 2.5   P = 3.0   F = 5

*Make holiday cookies with a cookie press.

½ cup butter or margarine, room temperature
½ cup shortening
4 cups cheddar cheese, finely grated
2-½ cups flour
½ teaspoon salt
½ teaspoon dry mustard
1 tablespoon chopped nuts

Preheat oven to 350 degrees. With mixer cream butter and shortening until well mixed and fluffy. Beat in cheese. Add ½ cup flour, salt and dry mustard beating until well mixed. Add remaining flour 1 cup at a time. When well mixed fill cookie press (or gun) and form cookies following directions for press on ungreased cookie sheet. Use nut piece to garnish centers of flowers or sprinkle on ribbons. Bake 9-11 minutes for medium thick shapes, checking early for thin cookie shapes and bake only until beginning to brown on edge. Cool carefully on wire rack.

* A bit of coloring in dough makes interesting holiday cookies!

# SPECIAL DESSERTS, GOODIES AND TREATS

## CRISPY MERINGUE DESSERT SHELLS

Serves 6
1 Serving Equals
Fruit Exchange Negligible
1/4 Lean Meat Exchange
9 Calories

C = .5  P = 1.75  F = 0

4 egg whites
1/2 teaspoon cream of tartar
1 teaspoon apple juice concentrate
1/2 teaspoon vanilla

Preheat oven to 275 degrees. Beat egg whites until foamy and soft peaks form. Add cream of tartar and beat until very stiff. Do not underbeat. Add apple juice concentrate and vanilla and continue beating until blended in. Divide mixture into six mounds on a lightly greased cookie sheet (or one lined with parchment paper) and shape mounds into 4 to 5 inch circular shells with a deep dent in the center of each. Bake approximately 45 minutes until firm to the touch and light brown. Remove from pan and cool on a wire rack. Fill right before serving.

Suggested Fillings — chopped or sliced fresh fruit, sugar free pudding, ice cream.

## STRAWBERRY SOUFFLE

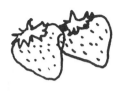

Serves 4
(Generously)
1 Serving Equals
½ Fruit Exchange
2 Fat Exchanges
Trace Lean Meat Exchange
129 Calories

C = 7.5  P = 1  F = 10.5

1 envelope unflavored gelatin
½ cup apple juice
2 teaspoons lemon juice
1-¼ cups unsweetened pureed strawberries
(about 1-½ cups strawberries if frozen berries are used)
2 egg whites
1 cup whipped cream

In small sauce pan heat apple juice and gelatin until gelatin dissolves. Remove from heat and add pureed berries and lemon juice. Stir to mix well. Chill, stirring occasionally, until mixture mounds slightly when dropped from a spoon. Beat egg whites until stiff but not dry. Fold egg whites in gelatin mixture. Next fold whipped cream in berry/egg white mix. Turn into a 3 cup souffle dish with a 2 inch collar or a 4 cup dish without a collar. Refrigerate at least 4 hours before serving.

*   May also be put in 4 individual souffle dishes.

*   Reserve two whole berries to cut in half and use for garnish.

*   For a light sweet treat divide equally into eight stemmed champagne glasses and garnish with a fresh berry. Cut values about in half for eight servings.

# PEACHES FLAMBE

Serves 4
1 Serving Equals
1 Fruit Exchange
Starch/Bread Negligible

2 cups (16 ounce can) peaches canned in fruit juice (room temperature)
¼ teaspoon cinnamon
1-½ teaspoons cornstarch
2 tablespoons warm brandy

Drain peaches and combine juice and cornstarch in a small pan. Cook over medium heat until thick and beginning to bubble. Stir in cinnamon. Add peach halves until just warm. Arrange peaches and sauce on serving platter. Pour on heated brandy and ignite. Serve flaming.

* This can be cooked in a large skillet tableside. Mix all ingredients except brandy and stir over flame with a peach half stuck on a fork (adds to the show). When thickened and fruit is warm, add the warm brandy and light.

* Alcohol evaporates when brandy is ignited.

* For Peaches Jubilee — serve over a scoop of low fat vanilla ice cream.

# PINEAPPLE "CHEATCAKE"

(A cheesecake with too few calories to believe!)
No crust — low calorie

Serves 8
1 Serving Equals
¾ Fruit Exchange
1 Fat Exchange
½ Medium Fat Meat Exchange
Milk Negligible
135 Calories

$C = 12 \quad P = 4 \quad F = 7.5$

1 20 ounce can pineapple in juice
1 envelope unflavored gelatin
½ cup skim milk
1 8 ounce package Neufchatel (cream-type) cheese
1 teaspoon vanilla
¼ teaspoon lemon juice
2 egg whites

Drain pineapple and reserve one cup of juice. (If there is not one cup add water to make one cup.) In a small sauce pan mix gelatin and milk. Cook over low heat about 2 minutes, stirring constantly, to dissolve gelatin completely. Remove from heat. In a large mixing bowl beat cheese until smooth and fluffy. Gradually beat in hot gelatin/milk mixture blending well. Next beat in the one cup pineapple juice, vanilla and lemon juice. Chill until mixture holds a kiss shape when dropped from a spoon. (about ½ hour). Beat egg whites until stiff. Fold egg whites and drained pineapple bits into cheese filling mixture. Turn into a 9 inch pie plate or spring form pan and chill until firm — 3 to 4 hours.

# FRESH STRAWBERRY SHORTCAKE

Serves 4
1 Serving Equals
1 Fruit Exchange
1 Bread Exchange
2 Fat Exchanges
230 Calories

C = 30  P = 3  F = 10

3-¾ cups fully ripe strawberries
⅓ cup unsweetened white grape juice or 8 teaspoons apple juice concentrate
4 2-½" diameter baking powder biscuits
½ cup whipped cream with vanilla to taste

Wash and slice or mash berries (leaving 4 whole for garnish). Mix the grape juice with the berries. Split the biscuits and spoon half the berries in the center – replace the top and add remaining berries. Top each shortcake with 2 tablespoons whipped cream. Garnish with whole ripe berry.

* Apple juice concentrate is sweeter.
* White grape juice provides more juice.

## RASPBERRY SHORTCAKE

Substitute 3 cups of fresh raspberries for strawberries. Values are the same as the strawberry shortcake.

# CREAM PUFFS

Makes 6
1 Puff Equals
½ Bread Exchange
⅓ Medium Fat Meat Exchange
2 Fat Exchanges
155 Calories

$C = 7.5$  $P = 3.5$  $F = 11.66$

½ cup water
¼ cup butter (½ cube)
½ cup flour
2 eggs

Heat water and butter to rolling boil in saucepan. Stir in flour and keep stirring until mixture forms a ball. Remove from heat and beat in eggs one at a time. Beat until smooth. Drop from spoon on ungreased cookie sheet. Bake at 400 degrees approximately 40 minutes. Shells should be puffed, dry and golden brown.

Cool away from drafts. Cut off tops and remove soft centers. Fill as desired.

* These are delicious when filled with whipped cream. For a special occasion sometimes fill them with a scoop of ice cream and top with chocolate sauce or strawberry topping.

* Custards and fresh fruit chunks mixed with whipped cream are also favorite fillings.

## CREAM PUFF SWANS

Make cream puffs above but reserve a small amount of batter to shape in 6 2" S shapes. Bake "S"s with shells. When cool and filling shells insert one S per puff for head. Fill and top with lid that has been cut in half to form 2 wings.

110

## CREAM PUFF WREATH

Serves 12
Values same as cream
puff servings

Make double cream puff recipe taking care to beat all 4 eggs in one at a time. Place in a circle on ungreased baking sheet with the 12 mounds about 1-½ – 1-¾ inches apart. Bake as directed. Dough will puff and edges touch. Carefully slit top off entire ring and fill as desired. Trim wreath with ribbon – holly – or pine boughs. Really a dessert-centerpiece in one!

* Good with a strawberry chiffon filling or berries folded in whipped cream. Festive and a light sweet ending.

## CUSTARD FILLING

Serves 6
1 Serving Equals
⅓ Milk Exchange
½ Medium Fat Meat Exchange
⅓ Fruit Exchange
85 Calories

$C = 9$  $P = 6.5$  $F = 2.5$

4 tablespoons cornstarch
2 cups skim milk
3 egg yolks
2 teaspoons vanilla
4 tablespoons apple juice concentrate, defrosted

Combine all ingredients. Cook over medium heat until mix thickens, stirring occasionally. Cool before filling desserts.

* Also makes good base for fruit topping and fruit parfaits.

## JIFFY PEACH COBBLER

Serves 6
1 Serving Equals
165 Calories
1 Bread Exchange
Milk negligible
⅔ Fruit Exchange
1 Fat Exchange

$C = 25 \quad P = 3 \quad F = 5$

1 16 ounce can sliced peaches in fruit juice
2 teaspoons tapioca
cinnamon to taste
1 cup biscuit mix
⅓ cup milk

Preheat oven to 350 degrees. Combine peaches and juice, tapioca and cinnamon in a 9" pie plate. Stir together biscuit mix and milk in small bowl and top fruit with 6 equal sized "mounds" of biscuit dough.

Bake 25-30 minutes.

* Serve warm with fruit dished on top of biscuit.
* Garnish with dollop of whipped cream if desired.
* Great breakfast treat.
* Quick dessert that cooks while eating dinner!

## JIFFY APRICOT COBBLER

Substitute 1 16 ounce can apricots for peaches and add 1 drop of almond extract. Values are the same as with peaches.

# CRAZY COBBLER

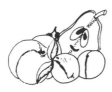

Serves 6
1 Serving Equals
1 Bread Exchange
Milk negligible
⅔ Fruit Exchange
1-⅓ Fat Exchange
180 Calories

C = 25  P = 3  F = 6.66

1 16 ounce can fruit cocktail in fruit juice
2 teaspoons tapioca
½ teaspoon cinnamon
1 cup biscuit mix
⅓ cup milk
¼ cup chopped nuts (large pieces)

Preheat oven to 350 degrees.
Combine fruit cocktail and juice, tapioca, cinnamon and nuts in a 9" pie plate. In small bowl stir together biscuit mix and milk. Drop biscuit dough on fruit in 6 equal mounds. Bake 25-30 minutes. Serve warm.

*  Good with milk or cream at breakfast.
*  Add a dollop of whipped cream and dessert in a jiffy!

# QUICK PEACH CRISP

Serves 4
1 Serving Equals
1 Fruit Exchange
¾ Bread Exchange
1 Fat Exchange
165 Calories

$C = 27$   $P = 2$   $F = 5$

2-¼ cups fresh peaches, peeled, pitted and sliced
2 tablespoons apple juice concentrate, thawed
1 tablespoon cornstarch
½ teaspoon cinnamon

Topping:
1 cup granola  (page 132)
2 teaspoons butter or margarine, melted

Preheat oven to 350 degrees. In a 4 cup baking dish (or 8 inch pie plate) combine peaches, apple juice concentrate, cornstarch and ½ teaspoon cinnamon. In a small bowl, combine granola, cinnamon and melted butter. Mix thoroughly to spread butter evenly through granola. Sprinkle granola mixture over peaches. Bake 30-35 minutes until thick and bubbly.

*   Delicious with a dollop of whipped cream.

## SPICY CINNAMON PEAR TWISTS

Topping
2 teaspoons melted butter
1 teaspoon cinnamon
3 tablespoons apple pear concentrate
5 tablespoons boiling water

2 fresh pears
1-½ cup flour
½ cup shortening
dash of salt
3 to 4 tablespoons cold water (for dough)

Serves 8
1 Serving Equals
(2 twists)
1-½ Bread Exchange
3 Fat Exchanges
½ Fruit Exchange
315 Calories

$C = 37.5 \quad P = 4.5 \quad F = 15$

Preheat oven to 450 degrees. Wash and core pears. Cut each pear into 8 slices. Set aside. Mix flour and salt in bowl. Add shortening and cut into flour until the size of peas. Add water and mix into a ball. Divide dough in half and roll each half out on a lightly floured pastry canvas into an 8 x 10 inch rectangle. Cut each rectangle into 8 (10" x 1") strips. Wrap one strip of dough around each pear wedge. Place in a 9 x 13 baking pan without touching. Brush with melted butter to which cinnamon was added. Mix water and concentrate and pour around pastries. Bake at 20-25 minutes until golden brown.

*   Excellent served warm with milk or cream.

## SPICY CINNAMON APPLE TWISTS

Substitute apples for pears and apple juice concentrate for apple-pear concentrate. Values remain the same as using pears.

# SIMPLE CREPES

1 cup pancake mix
1 cup skim milk
½ teaspoon almond extract
2 eggs

Makes 8
1 Starch/Bread Exchange
80 Calories

C = 15   P = 3   F = Trace
Add filling choice

Mix all ingredients with a wire whip in medium mixing bowl until smooth and free of lumps. Into a non-stick eight inch frying pan or crepe pan over medium heat spoon 3 tablespoons batter and move pan to have a thin film cover the bottom of the pan. Cook until beginning to firm through and brown the other sides. Continue until all batter is cooled — stacking crepes between paper towels to prevent sticking together. Fill and enjoy.

# BERRY FILLING

2 cups fresh raspberries or
2-½ cups fresh sliced strawberries
½ cup whipped cream (with a drop of vanilla)

Filling Only
Fills 8 Crepes
¼ Fruit Exchange
½ Fat Exchange
40 Calories

C = 4   P = 0   F = 2.5

Wash and drain fruit. Mix fruit with whipped cream and put ¼ cup of filling in each crepe. Roll and place seam side down. Top each with about two teaspoons remaining filling. Refrigerate until serving time.

# FRESH PEACH FILLING

* Use ½ cup whipped cream (with a drop of almond) and 2 cups sliced peaches. Values increase to ⅓ fruit exchange, ½ fat exchange, 45 calories  C = 5   P = 0   F = 2.5

# FRENCH PASTRY ICING

1 cube butter or margarine, room temperature
½ cup apple juice concentrate, defrosted
4-½ teaspoons flour
cinnamon, nutmeg, vanilla or almond extract
    to taste (takes a very small amount)

Makes 1-½ Cups
1 Serving Equals
2 Tablespoons
2 Fat Exchanges
⅓ Fruit Exchange
Starch/Bread negligible
125 Calories

$C = 7.5$  $P = .05$  $F = 10$

With wire whip blend apple juice concentrate and flour in small saucepan. Cook over medium heat until thick and glossy. Remove from heat and allow paste to cool completely. In a small mixing bowl beat butter until light and fluffy. Add thickened concentrate in 3 additions beating well. Season to taste. Spread on your favorite goodie.

* This icing may be thickened slightly and can be colored for a decorator icing.
* Orange and pineapple juice concentrates may be substituted for the apple for a flavor change.      * Very rich and sweet.

# CAROB GLAZE

1 tablespoon butter or margarine, room temperature
½ cup carob powder
7 tablespoons water
1 teaspoon vanilla

Makes about ¾ Cup

1 Teaspoon — negligible

Combine all ingredients in saucepan over medium heat. Cook, stirring occasionally until glaze thickens. Drizzle as desired. If glaze thickens too much before it is all used, just reheat slightly to return to "drizzle" consistency.

117

# ORANGE CREAM DESSERT

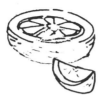

Serves 8
1 Serving Equals
Meat negligible
½ Fruit Exchange
2 Fat Exchanges
120 Calories

C = 7.5   P = 0   F = 10

2 cups unsweetened orange juice
1 envelope unflavored gelatin
1 drop almond extract
1 cup whipping cream (unwhipped)

Mix gelatin and ½ cup orange juice in small bowl and let set 2 minutes to soften. Boil remaining juice and add to gelatin mix and stir until dissolved. Refrigerate until thick and syrupy. Beat cream until light and fluffy. Add 1 drop almond to whipped cream and slowly add gelatin mixture to cream until just blended. Spoon into individual dessert dishes and refrigerate until set.

* May be refrigerated in a ring mold. Unmold and serve on platter with drained mandarin or fresh orange slices for garnish.
* Rich, elegant and tastes like the "old fashioned" cream-sicle!

## PINEAPPLE CREAM

Substitute pineapple juice for orange juice in orange cream dessert (or for a chunky dessert use juice packed crushed canned pineapple and juice as above). Values remain the same as Orange Cream Dessert.

118

# "GLORIFIED" CREAMY RICE PUDDING

Serves 6
One Serving Equals
1-⅓ Fat Exchanges
½ Fruit Exchange
1 Starch/Bread Exchange
180 Calories

C = 23  P = 3  F = 8

1 cup whipped cream
½ teaspoon vanilla
1 cup crushed pineapple*, well drained
2 cups cooked rice, cooled
dash of cinnamon

In a large bowl gently fold together whipped cream, vanilla and pineapple with a rubber scraper. Slowly add rice and mix gently. Spoon into custard cups and sprinkle lightly with cinnamon. Refrigerate one hour before serving. Store in refrigerator.

* One 16 ounce can of pineapple canned in pineapple juice yields approximately 1 cup crushed pineapple.

* Save juice – it's great to drink or for other recipes.

* Great use for leftover rice.

* Recipe may be cut in half to serve four. It is best the first day.

* Be sure pineapple is well drained or cream will separate and puddle.

# CHOCOLATE RUM PINEAPPLE SPEARS

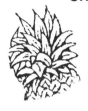

Makes 20 Spears
2 Spears Equal
One Serving
1 Fruit Exchange
Fat Negligible
65 Calories

1 fresh pineapple – cut into 20 (3 x ¾") spears
2 teaspoons rum flavoring (or to taste)
2 squares (1 ounce) semi-sweet chocolate
2 tablespoons orange juice

C = 15   P = 0   F = .5

Place pineapple spears in a single layer in a 9 x 13 inch dish and drizzle with rum flavoring. Cover and refrigerate 3-4 hours turning spears once. Remove from dish and pat dry with a paper towel. Set aside. Over low heat melt chocolate with orange juice (a double boiler over hot water is perfect) stirring constantly until chocolate melts. Dip each pineapple spear half way into chocolate mixture. Place on flat baking sheet in a single layer. Refrigerate until ready to serve and firm – about 2 hours. Carefully remove spears from baking sheet using a spatula. Arrange 2 spears on a plate and garnish with an orange slice or mint leaf.

# CHOCOLATE ORANGE SECTIONS

Peel an orange and separate sections leaving membranes intact. Dip sections half way into chocolate-orange juice mixture above and refrigerate until firm. 4 sections equal ⅓ fruit exchange, 20 calories  C = 5   P = 0   F = 0.

# SWEET STRAWBERRY ICE

Serves 5
1 Serving Equals
1 Fruit Exchange
60 Calories

C = 15  P = 0  F = 0

3-¾ cups fresh strawberries, hulled
¼ cup apple juice concentrate

Combine berries and juice in blender container.  Blend until smooth.  Pour mixture into an 8 inch square pan, cover and freeze until slushy.  Spoon mixture back into blender container and process until smooth.  Return to freezer and freeze until firm.

* Light sweet strawberry dessert.

* Slushy — this makes a terrific non-alcoholic frozen strawberrry cocktail.

## STRAWBERRY ICE

### (Tart Sweet)

Serves 4
1 Serving Equals
1 Fruit Exchange
60 Calories

C = 15  P = 0  F = 0

3-¾ cups fresh strawberries, hulled
½ cup unsweetened orange juice

Combine berries and juice in blender container. Blend until smooth.  Pour mixture into an 8 inch square pan, cover and freeze until slushy.  Spoon mixture back into blender container and process until smooth.  Return to freezer and freeze until firm.

* Tart-sweet ice is refreshing and good served with fruit.

* This ice is nice to serve in a small amount between dinner courses to cleanse the palate.

## FRESH STRAWBERRY SHERBET

Makes 1 quart
½ cup =
¾ fruit exchange
50 calories

C = 12.5  P = 0  F = 0

⅓ cup apple juice concentrate or fruit and berry concentrate
1 tablespoon lemon juice
½ cup water
5 cups fresh strawberries

Wash and stem berries. In a blender container combine concentrate, water and lemon juice. Add half the berries. Cover and blend until smooth. Add remaining berries and continue blending until smooth. Pour into a 9 x 13 inch pan, cover and freeze until firm. Scoop mixture into mixing bowl and beat with a mixer until smooth. Put in freezer container and freeze.

## BLACKBERRY SHERBET

Makes 1 quart
½ cup =
1 fruit exchange
60 calories

C = 15  P = 0  F = 0

Exchange fully ripe blackberries for strawberries above. This will be a bit more dense due to the type berries. Wonderful flavor.

# PINEAPPLE ICE

Serves 4 Generously
1 Serving Equals
1 Fruit Exchange
Lean Meat negligible
65 Calories

$C = 15 \quad P = 1 \quad F = trace$

1-½ teaspoons unflavored gelatin (½ envelope)
1 cup pineapple juice (canned — fresh will not set up)
1 tablespoon lemon juice
1 cup canned crushed pineapple in juice undrained
1 egg white, stiffly beaten

Mix gelatin, pineapple juice, lemon juice and pineapple in sauce pan. Bring to a full boil. Remove from heat and allow to cool. Pour into freezer tray (ice cube tray with grid network works well) and allow to freeze until mushy. Remove from freezer and beat until fluffy. Fold in beaten egg white. Freeze until firm, stirring twice.

## STRAWBERRY-PINEAPPLE OR RASPBERRY-PINEAPPLE ICE

May substitute 2-½ cups crushed strawberries or 2 cups raspberries for the cup of crushed pineapple for an interesting change. Values are the same as for Pineapple Ice.

# LOW CALORIE BERRY SHERBET

Serves 4 Generously
1 Serving Equals
½ Fruit Exchange
¼ Skim Milk Exchange
52 Calories

$C = 10.5$  $P = 2$  $F = trace$

1 cup skim or very low fat milk
2 tablespoons apple juice concentrate
Choice of berry (**one** from list)
1-¼ cup strawberries **or**
1 cup raspberries
(or) ¾ cup blackberries.

Pour milk into ice cube tray (divided type) and freeze until solid (2 to 3 hours). Refrigerate or freeze clean berries.  Shortly before serving, remove frozen milk cubes and berries (if frozen) and let stand at room temperature about 5 minutes.  Place cubes (about ⅓ at a time) in blender and process until chunky.  Add berries and process until smooth sherbet consistency.  Serve immediately or put into a freezer container with a tight lid and freeze to desired firmness. If sherbet is frozen solid remove from freezer and let stand at room temperature about 15 minutes before serving.

* If you do not have a blender, break up milk cubes with a wooden spoon and proceed as above using an electric mixer.  You may want to start on low speed and work up to high.  This will be a bit "chunkier" but just as tasty.

# LIGHT PINEAPPLE-PAPAYA SORBET

Serves 4
1 Serving Equals
½ Fruit Exchange
30 Calories

C = 7.5  P = 0  F = 0

½ cup pineapple juice
1 cup papaya, peeled and seeded
1 tablespoon lime or lemon juice

Combine all ingredients in blender or food processor and whirl until a smooth puree. Pour into a freezer container (a flat 9" cake pan works great). Cover and freeze until nearly firm (1-½ to 2 hours). Remove from freezer and put mix into a medium mixing bowl. Beat until slushy. Spoon sorbet into freezer container, cover tightly, and freeze until firm (about 2 hours). Scoop out and enjoy. Best if allowed to sit at room temperature 5-10 minutes before serving.

* Will keep tightly covered up to a month.

* For a smoothier sorbet – the mix can be poured through a fine strainer to remove any fibers before the first freezing.

* This can be processed in an electric or hand cranked ice cream maker. Process according to manufacturer's directions. This is my favorite way and when using the ice cream maker I double the recipe since it keeps well.

# TUTTI FRUITY ICE

Serves 36
½ Cup Serving
1 Serving Equals
1 Fruit Exchange
60 Calories

C = 15  P = 0  F = 0

2 (16 ounce) cans apricots in fruit juice
5 large (9 inch) very ripe bananas
3 cups cold water
1 (15 ounce) can crushed pineapple in juice
1 (12 ounce) can orange juice concentrate

Mash apricots in juice well with potato masher or puree in blender. Mash bananas. Pour all ingredients in electric or hand crank ice cream freezer and process according to manufacturers directions. Let ripen 1-2 hours before serving.

* Makes a gallon – great for a picnic.

* Will keep in freezer 2-3 weeks.

* I like to let the ice set at room temperature 10-15 minutes before serving.

"Taste spoons" while cooking are filled with calories that count!

# QUICK APPLE (PLUM) DESSERT

Serves 9
1 Serving Equals
1 Bread Exchange
1 Fruit Exchange
140 Calories

C = 31   P = 3   F = Trace

*If desired – 1 tablespoon whipped cream per serving adds 25 calories – 2.5 g. fat.

2 cups fully ripe plums, pitted and chopped
2 medium apples, sliced and peeled
¼ cup apple juice concentrate
2 tablespoons cornstarch or tapioca
¼ teaspoon cinnamon
1-½ cups biscuit mix
½ cup skim milk

Mix plums, apples, apple juice concentrate, cinnamon and cornstarch or tapioca in 8" square pan.  Mix milk and biscuit mix and drop in 9 equal mounds on fruit.  Bake at 350 degrees for 30-40 minutes until biscuits are lightly brown and fruit is tender and thickened.

Delicious warm with a tablespoon of whipped cream.

Pretty served in wine or stem type glasses.

Great for dessert or a real brunch treat.

# APPLE NUT SQUARES

Serves 8
1 Serving Equals
Meat negligible
¾ Fruit Exchange
½ Fat Exchange
55 Calories

C = 10   P = 0   F = 2.5

1 6 ounce can unsweetened apple juice concentrate, thawed
½ cup boiling water
3 envelopes unflavored gelatin
½ cup chopped walnuts or pecans

Place half apple juice concentrate in small bowl with gelatin. Let rest one minute to soften gelatin. Stir in boiling water mixing until gelatin is dissolved. Add remaining juice and nuts. Pour into a loaf pan and chill until firm. Cut into 16 bars. Store in refrigerator.

* These crunchy little candy squares with a gum drop consistency stay firm for a lunch box treat.
* Nuts will be mostly on top. For nuts mixed throughout refrigerate juice/gelatin mix, and stir in nuts.

# "GUMDROP" FRUIT CHEWS

Makes 64 Squares
4 Squares Equals
¼ Fruit Exchange
15 Calories

C = 3.75  P = 0  F = 0

Orange Pineapple Chews
4 envelopes gelatin
1 cup canned unsweetened pineapple juice
1 cup orange juice
¾ cup boiling water

In medium bowl mix gelatin with pineapple juice. Let rest 2 minutes to soften gelatin. Add boiling water and stir until gelatin is dissolved. Stir in cold orange juice. Pour into 8 inch pan and chill until firm. Cut into 1" squares to serve.

## GRANOLA BARS

Serves 8
2 Bars Equal
1 Fruit Exchange
½ Bread Exchange
1 Fat Exchange
145 Calories

C = 22.5  P = 1.5  F = 5

2 cups apple juice
2 cups granola
5 envelopes gelatin

Soften gelatin in ⅔ cup juice in mixing bowl. Boil one cup juice and stir in gelatin/juice. Continue stirring until gelatin dissolves. Add remaining cup of juice and stir in granola. Pour into 8" saucepan. Chill until set. Cut into 16 bars.

* Great for snacks, picnics or lunch boxes.
* Quick energy on the go!

## BASIC SWEET "GUMDROP" CHEW

Apple Chews – 5 Squares
Grape Chews – 4 Squares
Orange Chews – 5 Squares
Equal ½ Fruit Exchange
30 Calories

C = 7.5  P = 0  F = 0

3 cups apple juice, grape juice or orange juice
5 envelopes gelatin

Soften gelatin in 1 cup fruit juice in mixing bowl. Bring 1 cup juice to a boil and stir in gelatin/juice mix. Continue stirring until gelatin is dissolved. Add remaining cup of juice. Pour into 8" square pan and refrigerate until firm. Cut into 1" squares to serve.

* Red grape juice makes great chews.
* For a festive touch – cut squares with cookie cutter into holiday shapes – orange pumpkins – red hearts, etc.

## GUM DROP CHEWS

Free Food

C = 0
P = 0
F = 0

1 can fruit flavored diet soda
1/2 cup lemon juice
1/2 teaspoon vanilla
Artificial sweetener to equal 1/4 cup sugar (if desired)
5 envelopes unflavored gelatin
3-4 drops food coloring will give brighter festive chews

Mix half can soda and all other ingredients in small mixing bowl. Boil remaining soda and add to mixture until gelatin is dissolved. Pour into 8 x 8 baking dish and refrigerate until firm. Cut into squares. Orange is our family favorite.

# SNACKS

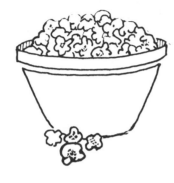

## SNACKERS MIX

Makes 16 Cups
1 Cup Equals
¼ Bread Exchange
1 Fat Exchange
1 Fruit Exchange
125 Calories

C = 19  P = 1  F = 5

3 quarts popped popcorn
1 cup salted nuts
1 cup raisins
1 cup fresh shredded coconut (not sugared)
1 cup sunflower seeds

Pop corn without fat and allow to cool. Mix in remaining ingredients. Store in airtight container.

* This is good to pack in 1 cup amounts in individual sandwich bags for camper and hiking snacks. Goes great in a back-pack!

* Super idea for classroom snack treats.

# GRANOLA

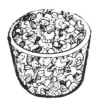

Makes 3 Cups
½ Cup Equals
1-½ Bread Exchange
1 Fat Exchange
⅓ Fruit Exchange
185 Calories

$C = 27.5$   $P = 4.5$   $F = 5$

2-¼ cups rolled oats (quick cooking kind are most tender)
¼ cup coconut, flaked or shredded unsweetened
¼ cup coarsley chopped nuts
2 tablespoons sunflower seeds
¼ cup raisins
1 teaspoon cinnamon

Preheat over to 350 degrees. Combine oats, coconut, nuts, and sunflower seeds on a non-stick baking pan. Bake uncovered until crisp and lightly browned — about 20 minutes. Stir every 5-8 minutes while in the oven to brown evenly. Cool completely and store in an airtight container.

* Great snack.

* Good with fresh peaches and milk for breakfast!

# TORTILLA CHIPS

8 Pieces = 1 Serving
1 Serving = 70 Calories
1 Bread Exchange

1 package corn tortillas
salt

$C = 15$   $P = 2$   $F = 0$

Cut each tortilla into 8 pie shaped wedges. Spread the pieces on a cookie sheet and sprinkle lightly with salt. Bake them at 400 degrees for about 8 minutes. Remove from the oven and with tongs or a pancake turner turn each one over. Bake for 3-4 more minutes. Cool on paper towels. Great with dips, salads and for a crunchy snack! A fat-free munchy.

Taco flavored seasoning gives a flavor of Old Mexico. Sometimes I use it instead of salt.

# POPCORN

Corn popped in an air popper pops without fat and contains only 80 calories in 3 cups popped and C = 15 grams, protein = 3 grams and fat = 0. Popcorn is satisfying and provides good bulk and roughage. Toppings are what make good popcorn great.

The following toppings sprinkled on popped corn are "free" and add nothing but flavor to your snack.

| | | | |
|---|---|---|---|
| garlic salt | taco seasoning | butter-flavored salt | bacon-flavored salt |
| curry powder | dried Italian herbs | dill weed | herb tea leaves |
| celery salt | hickory flavored salt | seasoned salt | (finely crushed) |
| chili powder | vegetable flakes | powdered orange rind | herb tea salt |
| | | | caraway seeds |

*3 cups of popcorn is more than 2 hands can hold!

# KIDS SNACKIN' CORN

1 Cup Equals 70 Calories
⅓ Bread Exchange
⅓ High Fat Meat Exchange
⅓ Fat Exchange

$C = 5$  $P = 3$  $F = 4.5$

9 cups popped corn
1 tablespoon butter or margarine
⅓ cup peanut butter

Pop the corn. This recipe is calculated on corn popped in an air type popper without added fat for fewer calories.

Over low heat melt the butter or margarine with peanut butter until runny. Drizzle over the popped corn and mix well. Spread in shallow baking pans and bake in 375 degree oven for 10 minutes stirring 2 or 3 times. The corn will crisp and topping will set.

Cool and enjoy.
Good for lunch crunchies and snacks.
Makes 9 cups.

\* To pop corn without fat an air popper is best. An electric popper or deep pan with a non-stick surface will work. Simply spray popper or pan well inside with "no-fat" frying cooking spray. Add 4 or 5 unpopped kernels and heat on high until the "test" kernels pop. When they pop add ⅓ cup popping corn. Cover and shake popper or pan to keep popped corn from scorching. When popping stops remove lid immediately to release steam and pour into bowl. Season and enjoy.

# "PEANUT BUTTER and JELLY" SNACK SQUARES

Serves 3
¾ Cup Equals
1 Starch/Bread Exchange
⅓ High Fat Meat Exchange
115 Calories

C = 15   P = 5   F = 3

2-¼ cups cereal squares (Chex, Crispix, etc.)
1 tablespoon peanut butter (I prefer chunky)
½ teaspoon fruit flavored sugar free "jello" type powdered mix

Preheat oven to 275 degrees. In a small sauce pan over low heat melt peanut butter and stir in powdered gelatin. Pour over cereal and stir (easiest to stir with a rubber scraper) until cereal is evenly coated. Bake 30 to 40 minutes stirring every ten minutes until cereal is crisp dry. Remove from oven and allow to cool. Store in an airtight container.

* This recipe may be doubled or tripled to make a larger batch.

* Strawberry and raspberry flavors are sweetest.

* Orange is tangy.

# NIBBLE MIX

Serves 8
1 Serving Equals
1 Bread Exchange
2 Fat Exchanges
170 Calories

C = 15  P = 3  F = 10

2 quarts popped corn
2 cups thin pretzel sticks
2 cups baked cheese korn-type curls
¼ cup butter or margarine
1 tablespoon worcestershire sauce
¾ teaspoon garlic salt

Preheat oven to 250 degrees. In 9 x 13 baking dish mix popped corn, pretzels and cheese curls. Melt butter in small saucepan adding worcestershire sauce and garlic salt. Drizzle over popped corn mix and stir well. Bake 45 minutes stirring 5 times to mix during cooking time.

*   Store leftovers – cool – in airtight containers.

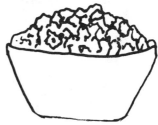

**Fun on a picnic . . .**

## POPCORN ON A STICK

Cook on a stick – eat from the pouch.

Makes 1 Serving
Equalling
1 Fat Exchange
½ Bread Exchange
85 Calories

C = 7.5  P = 1.5  F = 5

1 teaspoon oil
1 tablespoon popcorn, unpopped
salt to taste
1 square heavy aluminum foil 12'

Place oil and unpopped corn in center of foil, twist edges together to make a loose pouch. Attach pouch to stick with wire, string or folding foil edges together on the stick. Hold over hot coals (or can set on bar-b-que grill). Begin shaking gently as soon as corn starts to pop. When popped, remove from stick, open top of pouch taking care not to be burned on hot escaping steam. Salt to taste and enjoy!

## CAMPFIRE POPCORN

Place packet above on grill over hot coals until popped. Remove as soon as finished popping. Carefully open packet allowing steam to escape. Season to taste.

* It's amazing how popcorn cooked outside always tastes great around the campfire, blackened kernels and all!

## CAMPFIRE TOASTIES

1 tube (8 ounces) refrigerator biscuits
sticks
hot coals

Makes 20 Toasties
1 Toastie = 40 Calories
½ Bread Exchange

C = 7.5  P = 1.5  F = negligible

Open biscuits. Cut biscuit dough in half and stretch (like gum) until about 7 inches long. Wrap biscuit in a single layer around the end of a stick. Slowly roast over fire until biscuit puffs up and browns. These are loads of fun to do and so much safer than sticky marshmallows.

* It's fun to flatten and fill with a bit of cheese, sugar-free jelly or fruit bits before roasting. Be careful. Surprise fillings get **hot**. (Fillings count... add in what you use.)

*COOK-OUT FUN*

## FOIL ROASTED CAMP FIRE APPLES

6 small apples
2 tablespoons raisins
2 teaspoons cinnamon or apple pie spice
1 tablespoon butter or margarine

Serves 6
1 Serving Equals
1-1/6 Fruit Exchange
½ Fat Exchange
92 Calories

C = 17.5 P = 0  F = 2.5

Core apples, cut off collar and scoop out some of the flesh. Place each apple on an individual square of heavy duty aluminum foil. Fill each apple with one teaspoon raisins, ½ teaspoon spice and top with ½ teaspoon butter or margarine. Wrap packages tightly, sealing at the top. Bake on coals approximately 40 minutes until apples are tender.

* New cans of spice are stronger than ones that have been open a while – so use new spices sparingly.

# BEVERAGES

## THE SOCIAL SPIRIT

Alcohol is a source of many "hidden" calories (7 per gram) and is essentially void of other nutrients. Beer and wine contain carbohydrates in addition to the alcohol and all this must be figured into the diet.

Enjoy the spirit of socializing without the "spirits." There are "non-alcoholic" bar beverages that have real names, look like their spirited cousins, taste much like their alcoholic counterpart and fit into a modified diet.

A Greyhound is grapefruit juice and gin. Simply order the Virgin Greyhound and you'll get a glass of grapefruit juice. If a Greyhound comes with a slice of lime, the Virgin Greyhound will too. To you it's a savings of about 135 calories as 1-1/2 ounces of gin is equal to 3 fat exchanges. Count the grapefruit juice in your diet — 1/2 cup contains 60 calories, 1 fruit exchange.

Virgin Mary is brunch perfect. A Bloody Mary without vodka. 6 oz. is only 35 calories. If you want lemon with your tomato juice ask for Virgin Mary with a twist of lemon. Virgin Mary can be ordered with or without salt on the edge of the glass. Another option — simply order Virgin Mary with the celery and you're sure to get the crunchy celery stock to stir your juice and chew on. It's better to chew on the celery than be tempted by cocktail peanuts!

Orange juice is the base for a Screwdriver. A Virgin Screwdriver is just plain o.j. Virgin Drivers usually are served on the rocks (over ice) without asking. One half cup unsweetened orange juice is 60 calories, 1 fruit exchange.

If a drink has a name it is somehow "socially acceptable," booze or not. No one notices that what you order is "different" if it has a bar name. Plain tomato juice is different — Virgin Mary is social. Try it, it's fun, legal and — not only will you stay with your diet program — you'll know what a good time you've had! Cheers!

## TROPICAL ICE  TEA

Serves 2
1 Serving Equals
1 Fruit Exchange
60 Calories

C = 15  P = 0  F = 0

3 cups brewed tea
¾ cup pineapple juice, unsweetened
2 pineapple spears

Combine tea and pineapple juice and pour over ice.  Garnish with the pineapple spear
"stir stick."

## MINTED ICE TEA

Serves Two
One Serving Equals
1 Fruit Exchange
60 Calories

C = 15  P = 0  F = 0

2 cups brewed mint tea
1 cup pineapple juice, unsweetened

Combine tea and pineapple juice and pour over ice.  Garnish with lemon slice or mint leaves.

# CRANBERRY CHILL

Serves One
1 Serving Equals
1 Fruit Exchange
60 Calories
C = 15  P = 0  F = 0

⅓ cup cranberry juice
½ cup Sugar-Free 7-Up or lemon lime soda

Mix juice and Seven-Up or lemon lime soda and serve in a tall glass over ice. Garnish with a lemon slice.

# STRALADA

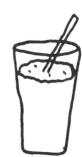

Serves Two
One Serving Equals
¾ Fruit Exchange
½ Fat Exchange
70 Calories
C = 12  P = 0  F = 2.5

¾ cup fresh or frozen strawberries, unsweetened
½ cup pineapple juice
2 tablespoons coconut cream
½ cup ice cubes

Place all ingredients in blender and blend until frothy. A delicious non-alcoholic combination of strawberry margarita and pina colada. Pour into a tall glass or snifter and garnish with a pineapple chunk or fresh strawberry.

# "MY" TAI

Serves 2
1 Serving Equals
1 Fruit Exchange
60 Calories

$C = 15$  $P = 0$  $F = 0$

¾ cup pineapple juice
¼ cup orange juice
1 tablespoon lime juice
¼ teaspoon rum extract (or to taste)
Crushed ice
Lime slices (optional)

Fill two (6 to 8 ounces) on the rocks glasses with ice. Combine all ingredients and pour over ice. Garnish with lime slice if desired!

# "MY" TAI LIGHT

Serves 4
1 Serving Equals
½ Fruit Exchange
30 Calories
$C = 7.5$  $P = 0$  $F = 0$

Make "My" Tai above adding 1 cup club soda or mineral water. Garnish with lime slices.

## ALOHA LITE

½ cup unsweetened pineapple juice
¼ to ½ cup mineral water

Serves One
1 Fruit Exchange
60 Calories

C = 15   P = 0   F = 0

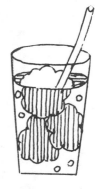

Pour over ice and garnish with an orange slice or pineapple chunk.

## ALOHA COOLER

½ cup unsweetened pineapple juice
½ cup Diet 7-Up or lemon lime soda

Pour over ice in stemmed glass and garnish with a pineapple chunk or sprig of mint. Values the same as Aloha Lite.

## STRAWBERRY FROST

Serves One Generously
1 Serving Equals
1-½ Fruit Exchange
95 Calories

C = 22   P = 0   F = 0

¾ cup fresh or frozen strawberries, unsweetened
½ cup orange juice, unsweetened
½ cup ice cubes

Place all ingredients in blender and blend until frothy.  Garnish.  Pour into tall glass and garnish with an orange slice or strawberry.

# NON-FAT PINA COLADA SMOOTHIE

Serves 2
1 Serving =
1 Fruit Exchange
1 Very Low Fat Milk Exchange
150 Calories

C = 27   P = 8   F = trace

⅔ cup crushed pineapple, canned in juice
1-½ cups very low fat or skim milk
2 tablespoons instant nonfat milk powder
¼ teaspoon coconut extract
1 teaspoon rum extract
4 ice cubes
2 small wedges of pineapple for garnish, optional

In blender container blend pineapple until smooth.  Add remaining ingredients except garnish and blend until frothy.  Pour into two glasses, garnish and serve.

*   I usually serve it with a straw so you can get all the foam off the sides.

*   If you do not want the rum flavor – omit rum and increase coconut extract to ½ teaspoon.

*   The crushed fruit and nonfat milk powder make the drink rich and thick.

# ORANGE SPICED TEA

4 cups boiling water
4 teaspoons loose tea or 3 tea bags
6-8 whole cloves
½ teaspoon dried orange peel
¼ teaspoon ground cinnamon (a bit less if can of cinnamon is new and strong)

Makes 4 Cups
1 Cup Free

C = 0   P = 0   F 0

Place spices and loose tea in tea ball or spice bag. Place in tea pot. Pour boiling water over tea ball or spice bag. Cover and let stand 3 to 5 minutes to desired strength. Remove tea ball or spice bag.

*   If tea bags are used follow above directions for spices only and place bags in pot. Shake spice bag while steeping for robust flavor.

## SPARKLING APPLE "BUBBLY"

Serves 6
1 Serving Equals
⅔ Fruit Exchange
40 Calories

C = 10   P = 0   F= 0

2 cups unsweetened apple juice, well chilled
2 cups (16 oz.) club soda, well chilled

Combine the chilled apple juice and soda. Serve in frosted or chilled wine glasses.

*   Great for any champagne occasion.

*   I like to garnish with one fresh strawberry.

# SPICED CIDER

3 cups apple cider
1 cup water
1 cinnamon stick
½ teaspoon whole cloves
½ teaspoon whole allspice
Orange and lemon slices for garnish
Cinnamon sticks (optional)

Makes 4 cups (8 servings)
½ cup =
¾ Fruit Exchange
45 Calories

C = 12   P = 0   F = 0

Simmer cider, water and spices together in saucepan for 10 minutes. Strain, if spices were not put in garni bag. Serve hot with fruit slice garnish and cinnamon sticks, if desired.

*   In punch bowl, top with baked clove-studded oranges.

ENJOY!

# SPICY SPRITZER

Serves 8
1 one cup serving equals
¾ Fruit Exchange
45 Calories

C = 12   P = 0   F = 0

Prepare spiced cider above and chill. At serving time add one half cup soda water or one half cup sparkling mineral water to one half cup spiced cider. Serve chilled in a wine glass or over ice in a tall beverage glass.

Refreshing!

A great way to user "left over" spiced cider.

# JIFFY GOODIES
# WITH NUTRA SWEET

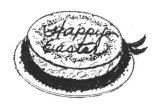

## BEST EVER FROSTING

Serves 12
1 Serving Equals
1 Fat Exchange
1/3 Starch/Bread Exchange
70 Calories

1 small package sugar free pudding mix
1 cup skim milk
1 small container Cool Whip, thawed

$C = 5$  $P = 1$  $F = 5$

Mix pudding mix and milk. Refrigerate 5 minutes until thick but not set. Fold in Cool Whip until well blended. Frosts an angel food cake generously. Refrigerate cake until serving time. Keep left overs refrigerated.

* Lemon and chocolate are our favorites!

* Caution . . . this is so good . . . but only one finger lick is free . . . all others count.

## BANANA CREAM PIE

Serves 6
(with crust)
1-1/16 Starch/Bread Exchanges
1 Fat Exchange
1/3 Fruit Exchange
150 Calories

1 Graham Cracker Crust (page 66 )
1 banana (9" long)
1 small package instant sugar-free vanilla pudding mix
2 cups skim milk

$C = 22.5$   $P = 3.5$   $F = 5$

Slice banana into bottom of cooled crust.  Make pudding according to the directions on the box.  Pour into graham cracker crust over the banana slices.  Refrigerate 2 hours before serving.  Party perfect with a dollop of whipped cream or whipped topping.

## CHOCOLATE CREAM PIE

Serves 6
(including crust)
1-1/16 Starch/Bread Exchanges
1 Fat Exchange
130 Calories

$C = 17.5$   $P = 3.5$   $F = 5$

1 Graham Cracker Crust (page 66 )
1 small package sugar-free chocolate pudding mix
2 cups skim milk

Make pudding according to the directions on the box.  Pour into cool graham cracker crust.  Refrigerate at least 2 hours before serving.  Enjoy!  Delicious with a dollop of whipped cream or whipped topping.

## NO-BAKE FRESH STRAWBERRY PIE

Serves 6
One Serving Equals
½ Bread Exchange
1 Fat Exchange
⅓ Fruit Exchange
100 Calories

C = 12.5  P = 1.5  F = 5
*Includes Crust

1 Graham Cracker Crust (page 66 )

½ package sugar free strawberry gelatin (4 serving size)
1 cup boiling water
2-½ cups fresh strawberries, hulled

Mix boiling water with the contents of half a package of the sugar free gelatin and stir continuously until dissolved. Refrigerate until slightly thickened but still pourable. Remove stems and hulls from fresh berries and arrange in graham cracker crust.  Spoon gelatin (You can't pour it easily as the berries will roll out!) to glaze and cover the strawberries. Refrigerate until firm.  This pie must be stored in refrigerator or it will get soggy.

*  Delicious with a dollop of whipped topping.

149

# NO-BAKE PEACH PIE

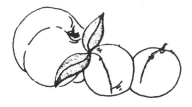

Serves 6
One Serving Equals
½ Bread Exchange
1 Fat Exchange
½ Fruit Exchange
115 Calories

C = 15  P = 1.5  F = 5
*Includes Crust

1 Graham Cracker Crust (page 66)

½ package sugar free lemon or pineapple gelatin (4 serving size)
1 cup boiling water
2-¼ cups sliced fresh peaches, peeled

Mix boiling water with the contents of half a package of the sugar free gelatin and stir continuously until dissolved. Refrigerate until slightly thickened but still pourable. Peel and slice peaches into graham cracker crust and pour gelatin mixture over fruit until peaches are covered with the glaze. Refrigerate until firm. Keep refrigerated until eaten to maintain fruit and consistency.

* For a spicy glaze I often add ¼ teaspoon of cinnamon to the gelatin powder before adding water.

# NO-BAKE BLACKBERRY PIE

Substitute fresh, fully soft-ripe blackberries for peaches in No-Bake Fresh Peach Pie. Values remain the same.

# STRAWBERRY ANGEL FOOD CAKE

(This cake makes any occasion a celebration.)

Serves 12
1 Serving Equals
2 Starch Exchanges
1 Fat Exchange
1/6 Fruit Exchange
215 Calories

C = 32.5  P = 6  F = 5

1 angel food cake
1 package (10 ounce) frozen unsweetened strawberries
1 cup boiling water
1 package (4 serving size) sugar free strawberry gelatin
1-½ cups whipped cream

Split angel food cake into 3 layers and set aside. In a medium mixing bowl combine gelatin and boiling water. Stir until gelatin is dissolved. Immediately add the frozen berries and continue stirring until berries are thawed and gelatin is partially thickened. Refrigerate until gelatin mix is soft set. With a rubber scraper gently fold whipped cream into berry gelatin until well mixed. Divide the berry whipped cream filling into thirds and put between each layer and on top. Refrigerate until serving time.

* I like to stack the cake back in my angel food pan. First I put in the bottom of the cake, then a filling layer, cake, more filling, cake and finally filling on top. I refrigerate in the pan until firm and cake is high, firm and pretty to serve when taken from refrigerated pan.

* This was my favorite birthday cake as a child.

# STRAWBERRY TOPPING

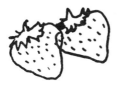

1/4 Cup = 1/4 Fruit
15 Calories

C = 4  P = 0  F = 0
1 Tablespoon Free

2 envelopes unflavored gelatin
1 can strawberry sugar-free pop
1 teaspoon lemon juice
2 cups strawberries
Artificial sweetener to equal 2 tablespoons sugar, if desired.

Wash and hull berries and set aside in strainer to drain. Mix gelatin and pop in sauce pan over medium heat until gelatin is dissolved. Add berries and lemon juice and simmer 5 minutes, stirring often. Add sweetener if needed. Crush berries with potato masher. Pour in covered container and refrigerate up to one week.

Great on pancakes, waffles, toast and ice cream treats. Makes about 2-1/2 cups.

* Raspberries and raspberry pop may be exchanged for strawberry.

# RASPBERRY-CUSTARD ICE MILK

Serves 12
(½ Cup Servings)
1 Serving Equals
⅓ Starch Exchange
Fruit Negligible
30 Calories
C = 5   P = 2   F = 0

3 cups very low fat milk
1 cup raspberries
1 package (4 serving size) instant sugar free pudding

Wash berries and crush thoroughly. Place berries, milk and pudding mix into container of hand or electric ice cream freezer and process according to directions for the ice cream maker.

This is wonderful immediately in the "soft serve" stage and delicious frozen. Freeze until firm. Stores up to 3 months.

\* Best if removed from the freezer 15 minutes prior to serving and allowed to soften a bit.

## FREEZER POPS

1 3-ounce cupful = 1 Serving
Serves 6
1 Serving = 5 Calories
Exchange Negligible

C = 0   P = 0   F = 0

1 package sugar-free flavored gelatin

Make as directed on package and pour into paper cups. Place in freezer until mushy (about 45 minutes). When mushy, put a wooden stick in each cup. Freeze until solid. Tear off cups and eat. Gelatin helps stop drips.

## POPSICLES/FLAVORED ICE CUBES

Free Exchange

Simply freeze diet soda or sugar-free punch in ice trays and add sticks. To stop the "drippys" I often heat soda with 1 tablespoon gelatin before freezing.

Try these ice cubes for color or as a "flavor savor" in cold beverages.

## JIFFY SNOW CONE

Place flavored ice cubes (above) in blender container. Cover and chop into snow. Slurp or eat with a spoon. Free exchange.

# JIFFY CHOCOLATE ICE CREAM

Serves 6
One Serving Equals
⅔ Starch/Bread Exchange
⅓ Milk Exchange
85 Calories
$C = 14$  $P = 5$  $F = 0$

1 package (4 serving size) instant sugar free chocolate pudding mix
3 cups skim milk

Combine sugar free pudding mix and skim milk and mix well. Pour into ice cream freezer container and freeze according to directions for ice cream freezer.

## EASY FUDGE POPS

Make Jiffy Chocolate Ice Cream above using chocolate fudge sugar free pudding mix instead of the chocolate. While soft set spoon into 6 (5 ounce) paper cups and put in a popsicle stick. Freeze until firm. Tear off paper cup before serving. These taste like old fashioned fudgesicles. Values are same as above.

* Tongue depressers from the drug store are great popsicle sticks and very inexpensive.

# INDEX

## Special Desserts, Goodies & Treats

## Beverages

## Snacks

## Nutra Sweet

## NOTES

# Other
# SUGAR FREE COOKBOOKS
## by
## Judith Soley Majors

### "Sugar Free... Goodies"   $7.95

Goodies Galore... all sweetened with fruit and fruit juice. Pies, cakes, bread, cookies, treats and much, much more. (Some of these goodies have won blue ribbons against sugared treats in various state fairs!)

### "Sugar Free... Kids' Cookery"   $6.95

Easy recipes for children that the entire family will enjoy! Calculated by calorie, exchange and CPF value. A variety of foods from breakfast to bed time snack. Approved by the American Diabetes Assn., Oregon Affiliate, Inc. Easy to read large red type. Also a favorite of senior citizens.

### "Sugar Free... Family Favorites"   $8.95

Calculated by calorie and exchange for any diet! Taste tempting foods and goodies without artificial sweeteners for your entire family. CPF figured for appetizers, main dishes, salads, snacks, pies, goodies and more... all fruit and fruit juice sweetened.

# Sugar Free Cookbook Order Form

Please send me:

_____ copies of Sugar Free... Good and Easy  $6.95
_____ copies of Sugar Free... Goodies ............ $7.95
_____ copies of Sugar Free... Kids' Cookery.... $6.95
_____ copies of Sugar Free... Family Favorites  $8.95
_____ copies of Sugar Free... Hawaiian Cookery $6.95

Please add $1.50 postage and handling.

Enclosed is my check or money order payable to APPLE PRESS for _____

Send to:

NAME_____

ADDRESS _____

CITY _____ STATE _____ ZIP _____

Mail Orders to: Apple Press
　　　　　　　　5536 S.E. Harlow
　　　　　　　　Milwaukie, Oregon 97222

Payment must accompany order. Specify if Gift Card to be enclosed. Prices subject to change.